VEGAN SIBO COOKBOOK

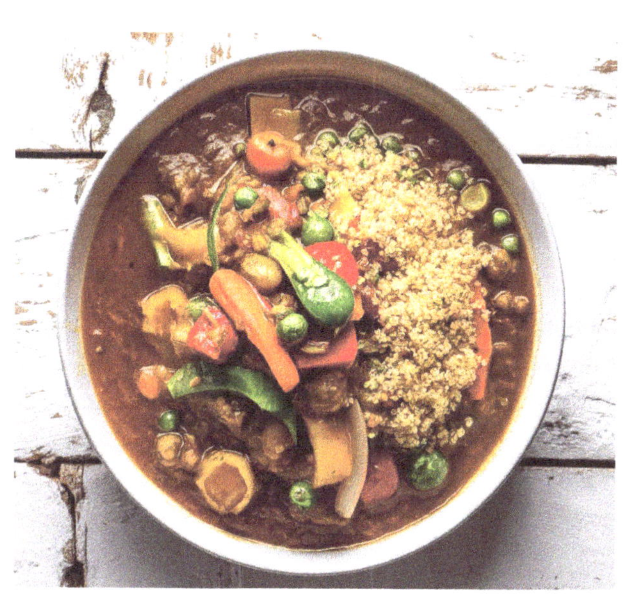

Delicious Plant-Based, Low-FODMAP Recipes for Managing Abdominal Pain and Other SIBO Symptoms

Esther Camara

Copyright © Esther Camara (2024)

The contents of this book are based on the author's research, knowledge, and experience. They are meant for educational purposes only and should not be taken as medical advice. Readers should consult their healthcare provider before making any changes to their health regimen.

Table of Contents

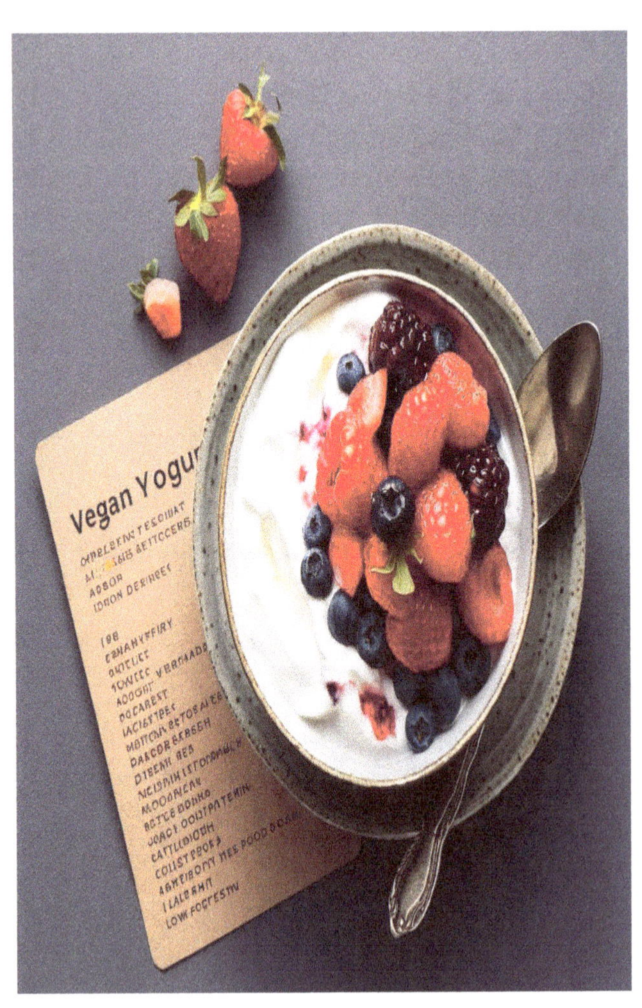
Vegan Yogurt

Introduction

When Uncle Peter first started complaining of feeling perpetually bloated after meals, we all brushed it off as "overindulging" at his favorite burger joint again. But the bloating never went away, and it escalated to gas, stomach cramps, and even fatigue. That's when the alarm bells went off for me – as a doctor and nutritionist, I knew these weren't just random digestive hiccups.

A battery of tests later, the culprit was identified: SIBO – Small Intestinal Bacterial Overgrowth. Basically, a party of unwelcome bacteria had crashed the small intestine, disrupting the delicate ecosystem there and causing all sorts of havoc.

Uncle Peter, a self-proclaimed "grill master," wasn't thrilled with the prospect of dietary changes. But trust me, the thought of endless bloating and discomfort was far less appealing. That's when I dug deep into the research and discovered the surprising ally in this battle: a vegan diet.

Now, I know what you're thinking – vegan and SIBO management? Sounds like a double whammy. But hear me out. A well-planned vegan diet is a powerhouse of fiber, which keeps things moving smoothly in the digestive system. Plus, it eliminates a lot of potential FODMAP triggers – those sneaky short-chain carbohydrates that can wreak havoc on a gut already under siege by SIBO.

The transition wasn't easy – there were definitely some "hanger" moments for Uncle Peter at first. But with some creative recipe swaps and a focus on delicious, gut-friendly whole foods, we turned things around. Within weeks, the bloating started to subside, the cramps became less frequent, and his energy levels skyrocketed. It wasn't just about managing SIBO; it was about feeling good again.

This book is a culmination of all that research, recipe experimentation, and most importantly, the success story of Uncle Peter. It's packed with delicious, low-FODMAP vegan recipes that are not only good for your gut but will tantalize your taste buds. So, if you're facing the frustration of SIBO, or just looking to give your gut a healthy boost, this book is your roadmap to feeling fantastic from the inside out. Let's get cooking!

Chapter 1: Understanding SIBO

Small Intestinal Bacterial Overgrowth (SIBO) is a digestive disorder where there's an unusual rise in the number or variety of bacteria in the small intestine. The small intestine, located between the stomach and large intestine, is primarily responsible for absorbing nutrients from food. A healthy small intestine maintains a specific balance of bacterial populations. However, in individuals with SIBO, this balance is disrupted, leading to a variety of digestive problems.

Symptoms of SIBO

* Bloating and abdominal discomfort
* Diarrhea or constipation
* Excessive gas
* Nausea and vomiting
* Abdominal pain and cramping
* Fatigue and weight loss (unintentional)

Causes of SIBO

The exact causes of SIBO are not fully understood, but several factors can contribute to its development:

- **Changes in gut motility**: Conditions that slow down the movement of food through the small intestine, such as irritable bowel syndrome (IBS), can allow bacteria to overgrow.
- **Surgery**: Abdominal surgeries that alter the anatomy of the digestive system can increase the risk of SIBO.
- **Antibiotics**: While antibiotics are used to treat bacterial infections, they can also disrupt the natural balance of gut bacteria, potentially leading to SIBO.
- **Underlying medical conditions**: Certain medical conditions like diabetes, scleroderma, and celiac disease can increase the risk of SIBO.

Diagnosing SIBO

There is no single definitive test for SIBO. Diagnosis often involves a combination of medical history, physical examination, and breath testing. Specific breath tests measure the amount of hydrogen or methane gas produced by gut bacteria after ingesting a sugar solution.

Types of SIBO

- **Hydrogen Dominant SIBO**: This is the most common type, where excessive hydrogen gas production is detected in the breath test. This type of SIBO is often associated with fermentation of simple sugars by bacteria.
- **Methane Dominant SIBO**: This type is characterized by an overgrowth of methane-producing bacteria. Methane gas can be more difficult to detect with breath tests, and other methods like stool testing may be needed for diagnosis.
- **Mixed SIBO**: This type involves an overgrowth of both hydrogen- and methane-producing bacteria.

Impact of SIBO on Gut Health

SIBO can significantly impact gut health by:
- **Interfering with nutrient absorption**: The overgrowth of bacteria in the small intestine can compete with the body for essential nutrients, leading to deficiencies.

- **Damaging the intestinal lining**: Chronic inflammation caused by SIBO can damage the lining of the small intestine, further hindering nutrient absorption.
- **Disrupting the gut microbiome**: The imbalance of bacterial populations in SIBO disrupts the natural gut microbiome, which plays a crucial role in digestion, immune function, and overall health.

Understanding SIBO and its impact on gut health is the first step towards managing this condition. The following chapters will explore the benefits of a vegan diet for managing SIBO symptoms, introduce the low-FODMAP approach, and provide delicious and nutritious vegan recipes to support your journey towards a healthier gut.

Chapter 2: The Vegan Approach to SIBO Management

For individuals diagnosed with SIBO, navigating dietary changes can feel overwhelming. This chapter explores the potential benefits of a vegan diet for managing SIBO symptoms and introduces the low-FODMAP approach as a valuable tool. We will also address essential nutrients for gut health within a vegan framework and provide tips for successfully combining a vegan lifestyle with SIBO restrictions.

Benefits of a Vegan Diet for SIBO

Several aspects of a well-planned vegan diet can be beneficial for individuals with SIBO:

- **High Fiber Content**: Plant-based foods like fruits, vegetables, legumes, and whole grains are naturally rich in fiber. Fiber promotes healthy gut motility, aiding in the movement of food through the digestive system and preventing bacterial overgrowth.
- **Reduced Inflammation**: Vegan diets tend to be lower in saturated fat and inflammatory compounds found in animal

products. This can help reduce inflammation in the gut, which is often a contributing factor in SIBO.

- **Prebiotic Powerhouse**: Many plant-based foods like legumes, fruits, and vegetables contain prebiotics, which are non-digestible fibers that serve as food for beneficial gut bacteria. Prebiotics help promote the growth of these good bacteria, fostering a healthier gut microbiome.
- **Dietary Diversity**: A well-planned vegan diet encourages a wider variety of fruits, vegetables, and whole grains. This diversity provides a broader range of nutrients and supports a more balanced gut microbiome compared to diets with limited food options.

Introducing the Low-FODMAP Diet

The low-FODMAP diet is a structured elimination and reintroduction approach designed to identify and manage food intolerances that can exacerbate digestive issues like those experienced with SIBO. FODMAP stands for Fermentable Oligosaccharides, Disaccharides, Monosaccharides, and Polyols - short-chain carbohydrates that are poorly absorbed in the small intestine and can contribute to bloating, gas, and other digestive discomfort.

While not a cure for SIBO, the low-FODMAP diet can be a valuable tool to identify specific FODMAPs that trigger your symptoms. By eliminating high-FODMAP foods for a period and then gradually reintroducing them, you can create a personalized eating plan that minimizes digestive distress.

Essential Nutrients for Gut Health in a Vegan Diet

Maintaining a healthy gut microbiome requires a good balance of essential nutrients. Here's how to ensure you get them on a vegan diet:

- **Protein**: Legumes like lentils, beans, tofu, and tempeh are excellent sources of plant-based protein. Seeds and nuts also contribute protein while providing healthy fats.
- **Healthy Fats**: Include sources like avocado, nuts, seeds, and olive oil in your diet for healthy fats that support gut health and nutrient absorption.
- **Iron**: Leafy greens, fortified plant milks, lentils, and tofu are good sources of iron, a crucial mineral for gut function.

- **Vitamin B12**: This vitamin is essential for nervous system function and can be challenging to obtain on a strict vegan diet. Consider fortified plant milks, nutritional yeast, or a vegan B12 supplement.
- **Probiotics**: Fermented foods like kimchi, sauerkraut, and tempeh contain beneficial probiotic bacteria that can aid digestion and gut health. Consider incorporating them into your diet.

Tips for Combining Vegan and Low-FODMAP

- **Read Labels Carefully**: Many processed vegan foods can contain hidden high-FODMAP ingredients. Always check labels for ingredients like wheat, dairy, certain fruits, and artificial sweeteners.
- **Focus on Whole Foods**: Base your diet on whole, unprocessed plant-based foods like fruits, vegetables, legumes, and whole grains. These are naturally low-FODMAP and provide essential nutrients for gut health.
- **Plan Your Meals**: Planning your meals in advance helps ensure you have low-FODMAP options readily available and

avoids impulse choices that might trigger symptoms.

- **Seek Guidance**: Consider consulting a registered dietitian familiar with both vegan diets and SIBO. They can help you create a personalized meal plan that addresses your specific needs and preferences.

By understanding the benefits of a vegan diet and incorporating the low-FODMAP approach, you can create a foundation for managing SIBO symptoms while embracing a healthy, plant-based lifestyle. The following chapters will provide delicious and nutritious vegan recipes that are low-FODMAP friendly, allowing you to explore culinary options that support your gut health journey.

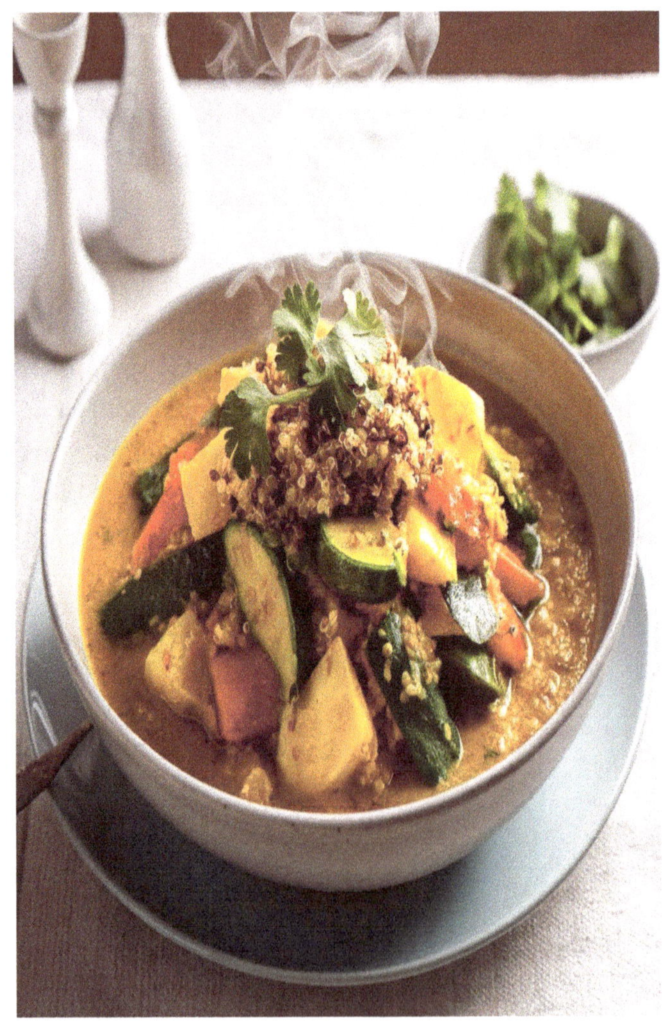

Chapter 3: Breakfast Recipes

Savory Chickpea Scramble

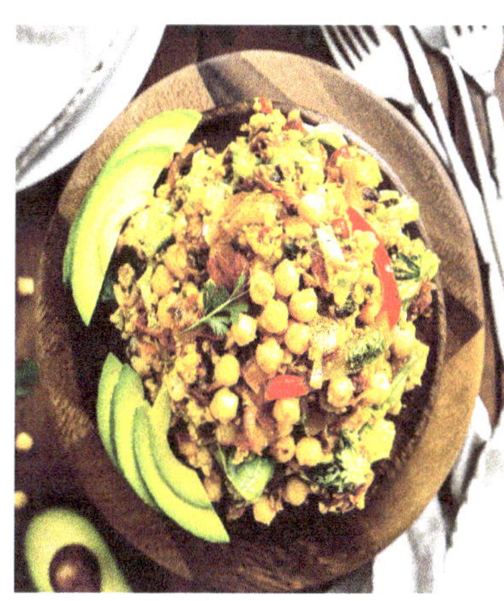

Preparation time: 5 minutes
Cooking time: 15 minutes
Servings: 2

Ingredients:
- 1 can (15 oz) chickpeas, rinsed and well-drained
- 1/2 cup chopped vegetables (bell pepper, mushrooms - choose low-FODMAP options)
- 1 tablespoon olive oil
- 1/4 teaspoon turmeric
- 1/4 teaspoon smoked paprika
- 1/4 teaspoon cumin
- Salt and pepper to taste
- Chopped fresh herbs (optional: parsley, cilantro)
- Vegan cheese (optional, choose low-FODMAP option)

Directions:

1. Warm olive oil in a pan over medium heat. Add chopped vegetables and cook until softened, about 5 minutes.

2. Mash half of the chickpeas with a fork. Add mashed and whole chickpeas to the pan with vegetables.

3. Stir in turmeric, paprika, cumin, salt, and pepper. Cook for another 5 minutes, breaking up the chickpeas with a spatula as desired.

4. Taste and adjust seasonings as needed.

5. Serve hot, topped with fresh herbs and vegan cheese (if using).

Nutritional value per serving (estimated):

Calories: 300   *Fiber: 10g*
Carbs: 40g   *Protein: 15g*
Cholesterol: 0mg   *Sodium: 250mg*
Total Fat: 10g

Notes:

- You can adjust the amount of vegetables and spices according to your preference.

- For a creamier texture, you can mash more chickpeas or add a splash of plant milk.

- This scramble can be served with toast, gluten-free wraps, or roasted vegetables.

Chia Seed Pudding

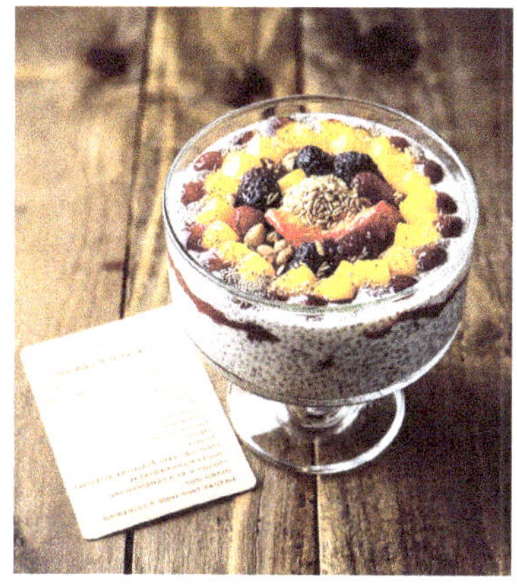

Preparation time: 5 minutes (plus overnight soaking)
Cooking time: N/A
Servings: 1

Ingredients:
- 1/4 cup chia seeds
- 1 cup unsweetened plant milk (almond milk, coconut milk)
- 1/2 teaspoon vanilla extract (optional)
- 1 tablespoon maple syrup (or your preferred sweetener)
- Toppings (fresh berries, chopped nuts, shredded coconut)

Directions:

1. In a jar or container, combine chia seeds, plant milk, vanilla extract (if using), and maple syrup. Stir well.

2. Cover and chill in the refrigerator for at least 4 hours, ideally overnight.

3. In the morning, stir the pudding again. The chia seeds will absorb the liquid and thicken.

4. Top with your favorite toppings and enjoy!

Nutritional value per serving (estimated):

Calories: 250   *Fiber: 10g*
Carbs: 25g   *Protein: 4g*
Cholesterol: 0mg   *Sodium: 30mg*
Total Fat: 10g

Notes:

- Adjust the sweetness and flavorings to suit your taste.

- Feel free to experiment with different types of plant milk and spices like cinnamon or ginger.

- The pudding will thicken more as it sits in the fridge.

Buckwheat Pancakes

Preparation time: 10 minutes
Cooking time: 15 minutes
Servings: 2-3 pancakes

Ingredients:
- 1/2 cup buckwheat flour
- 1/4 cup unsweetened plant milk (almond milk, oat milk)
- 1/4 cup sparkling water (or water)
- 1 tablespoon mashed banana (ripe)
- 1/4 teaspoon baking powder
- Pinch of salt
- Olive oil for cooking

Directions:
1. In a mixing bowl, whisk together buckwheat flour, plant milk, sparkling water (or water), mashed banana, baking powder, and salt.
2. Warm a lightly greased pan over medium heat.
3. Pour about 1/4 cup of batter per pancake onto the pan.
4. Cook for 2-3 minutes per side, or until bubbles appear on the surface and the edges begin to set.

5. Flip the pancakes and cook for another 1-2 minutes, or until golden brown.

6. Serve warm with your favorite toppings like fruit, maple syrup, or vegan butter.

Nutritional value per serving (estimated):

Calories: 200
Carbs: 30g
Cholesterol: 0mg
Total Fat: 5g

Fiber: 3g
Protein: 4g
Sodium: 60mg

Notes:

- You can enhance the batter's flavor by adding a pinch of ground cinnamon or nutmeg.

- If the batter seems too thick, add a splash more plant milk. If it's too thin, add a tablespoon more buckwheat flour.

- Buckwheat pancakes can be a bit delicate, so flip them carefully with a spatula.

- Leftover pancakes can be stored in an airtight container in the refrigerator for up to 2 days and reheated in a toaster or pan.

Coconut Yogurt Parfait

Preparation time: 5 minutes
Cooking time: N/A
Servings: 1

Ingredients:
- 1/2 cup unsweetened coconut yogurt (choose a low-FODMAP brand)
- 1/4 cup chopped fruits (berries like blueberries, raspberries, or chopped kiwi)
- 1/4 cup granola (choose a low-FODMAP option)
- Hemp seeds or chopped nuts (optional)

Directions:
1. In a parfait glass or bowl, layer the coconut yogurt, chopped fruits, and granola.
2. Repeat layers if desired.
3. Top with hemp seeds or chopped nuts for extra texture and nutrients (optional).
4. Enjoy chilled.

Calories: 300
Carbs: 30g
Cholesterol: 0mg
Total Fat: 10g

Fiber: 4g
Protein: 4g
Sodium: 60mg

Notes:

- You can use different types of low-FODMAP fruits for the parfait, such as chopped mango or sliced banana.

- Make sure the granola you choose is low-FODMAP and doesn't contain ingredients like wheat, high-fructose corn syrup, or inulin.

- This is a quick and easy breakfast option that can be customized according to your preferences.

Vegetable Frittata

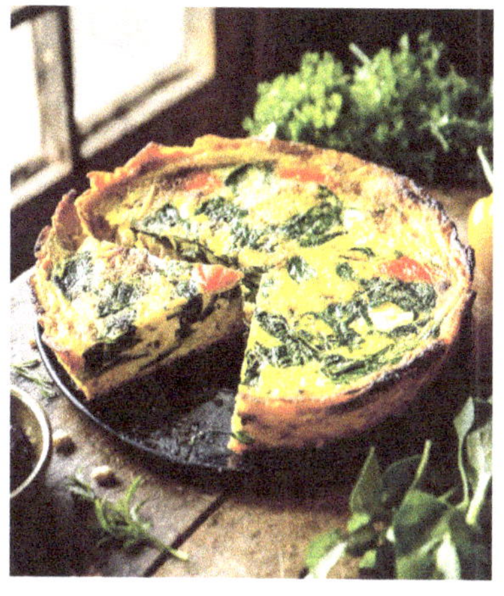

Preparation time: 10 minutes
Cooking time: 20-25 minutes
Servings: 2-3

Ingredients:
- 1 tablespoon olive oil
- 1/2 cup chopped vegetables (low-FODMAP options like zucchini, bell peppers, mushrooms, spinach)
- 1/4 cup chickpea flour (or another gluten-free flour blend)
- 1 cup unsweetened plant milk (almond milk, oat milk)
- 1/4 teaspoon turmeric
- 1/4 teaspoon dried herbs such as Italian seasoning or thyme
- Salt and pepper to taste
- Chopped fresh herbs (optional: parsley, cilantro)

Directions:

1. Preheat oven to 375°F (190°C). Grease a small oven-safe skillet or baking dish.
2. Warm olive oil in a pan over medium heat. Add chopped vegetables and cook until softened, about 5 minutes.
3. In a separate bowl, whisk together chickpea flour, plant milk, turmeric, dried herbs, salt, and pepper.
4. Pour the chickpea flour mixture over the cooked vegetables in the pan.
5. Gently stir to combine.
6. Transfer the pan to the preheated oven and bake for 20-25 minutes, or until the frittata is set and golden brown on top.
7. Let cool slightly before serving.
8. Top with chopped fresh herbs (optional).

Nutritional value per serving (estimated):

Calories: 250
Carbs: 30g
Cholesterol: 0mg
Total Fat: 10g

Fiber: 5g
Protein: 10g
Sodium: 200mg

Notes:

- You can experiment with different low-FODMAP vegetables in your frittata.

- If you don't have chickpea flour, you can try another gluten-free flour blend like oat flour or brown rice flour.

- Leftover frittata can be stored in an airtight container in the refrigerator for up to 3 days and reheated in a pan or microwave.

Green Smoothie

Preparation time: 5 minutes
Cooking time: N/A
Servings: 1

Ingredients:
- 1 cup unsweetened plant milk (almond milk, spinach milk)
- 1 handful of leafy greens (spinach, kale - choose low-FODMAP options)
- 1/2 banana (frozen or fresh)
- 1/4 cup berries (blueberries, raspberries)
- 1 scoop vegan protein powder (choose a low-FODMAP option)
- Optional: 1 tablespoon chia seeds, pinch of ginger

Directions:
1. Blend all ingredients together in a high-powered blender until smooth and creamy.
2. Add a splash more plant milk if needed to achieve desired consistency.
3. Enjoy immediately!

Nutritional value per serving (estimated):

Calories: 300
Carbs: 40g
Cholesterol: 0mg
Total Fat: 5g

Fiber: 5g
Protein: 20g
Sodium: 40mg

Notes:

- This recipe provides a good balance of protein, carbohydrates, and healthy fats to keep you feeling full and energized.

- You can adjust the sweetness of the smoothie by using more or less banana or adding a natural sweetener like stevia.

- Make sure the vegan protein powder you choose is low-FODMAP and free of ingredients like whey or soy protein isolate, which can be problematic for some.

- Chia seeds can add extra fiber and texture to the smoothie.

- Ginger can add a nice warming flavor and may have digestive benefits.

Tofu Scramble

Preparation time: 10 minutes
Cooking time: 15 minutes
Servings: 2

Ingredients:
- 1 block (14 oz) firm tofu, drained and pressed
- 1/2 cup chopped vegetables (low-FODMAP options like bell peppers, mushrooms)
- 1 tablespoon olive oil
- 1/4 teaspoon turmeric
- 1/4 teaspoon smoked paprika
- 1/4 teaspoon nutritional yeast
- Salt and pepper to taste
- Chopped fresh herbs (optional: parsley, cilantro)
- Vegan cheese (optional, choose a low-FODMAP option)

Directions:
1. Crumble the tofu with your hands or a fork into a bowl.
2. Warm olive oil in a pan over medium heat. Add chopped vegetables and cook until softened, about 5 minutes.
3. Add crumbled tofu to the pan with vegetables.

4. Stir in turmeric, paprika, nutritional yeast, salt, and pepper.

5. Cook for another 5-7 minutes, breaking up the tofu further with a spatula as desired.

6. Taste and adjust seasonings as needed.

7. Serve hot, topped with fresh herbs and vegan cheese (if using).

Nutritional value per serving (estimated):

Calories: 300

Carbs: 20g

Cholesterol: 0mg

Total Fat: 15g

Fiber: 2g

Protein: 20g

Sodium: 200mg

Notes:

- Pressing the tofu removes excess moisture, resulting in a drier and crumblier scramble.

- You can experiment with different low-FODMAP spices and herbs to customize the flavor of your scramble.

- Tofu scramble can be served with toast, gluten-free wraps, or roasted vegetables.

- Leftovers can be stored in an airtight container in the refrigerator for up to 2 days and reheated in a pan or microwave.

Seaweed Salad

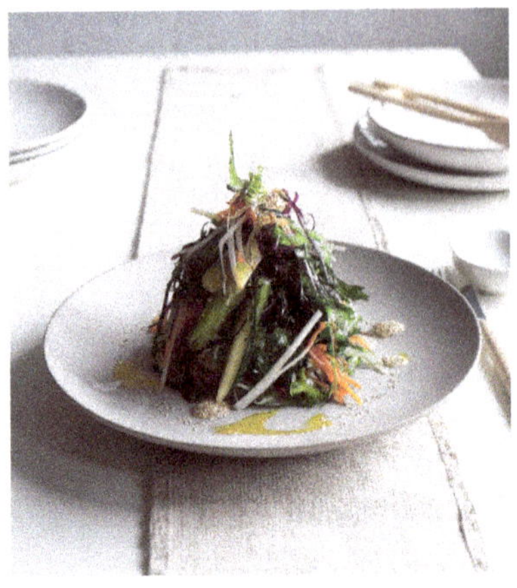

Preparation time: 10 minutes
Cooking time: N/A
Servings: 2

Ingredients:
- 1 package (2 oz) wakame seaweed, rinsed and drained
- 1 cucumber, thinly sliced
- 1 tablespoon rice vinegar
- 1 teaspoon sesame oil
- 1/2 teaspoon grated ginger (optional)
- Pinch of red pepper flakes (optional)
- Sesame seeds for garnish (optional)

Directions:
1. In a bowl, combine rinsed and drained wakame seaweed and sliced cucumber.

2. In a separate small bowl, whisk together rice vinegar, sesame oil, ginger (if using), and red pepper flakes (if using).
3. Pour the dressing over the seaweed and vegetables.
4. Toss gently to coat.
5. Garnish with sesame seeds (optional) and serve chilled.

Nutritional value per serving (estimated):

Calories: 50
Carbs: 5g
Cholesterol: 0mg
Total Fat: 1g

Fiber: 2g
Protein: 2g
Sodium: 150mg

Notes:
- You can find wakame seaweed in most Asian grocery stores or online.
- Feel free to adjust the amount of dressing or red pepper flakes to your taste preference.
- This is a light and refreshing salad that is perfect as a side dish or appetizer.

Roasted Sweet Potato Toast

Preparation time: 10 minutes
Cooking time: 40-45 minutes
Servings: 2

Ingredients:
- 1 large sweet potato
- 1/4 cup mashed avocado
- Chopped fresh herbs (optional: cilantro, parsley)
- Hemp seeds or chopped nuts (optional)
- Salt and pepper to taste

Directions:
1. Preheat oven to 400°F (200°C). Place parchment paper on a baking sheet.
2. Wash and slice the sweet potato into thick rounds (about 1/2 inch thick).
3. Arrange the sweet potato slices on the prepared baking sheet.
4. Bake for 30-40 minutes, or until tender and slightly crispy on the edges. Flip the slices halfway through baking for even cooking.
5. While the sweet potato is baking, mash the avocado in a bowl. Season with salt and pepper to taste.

6. Once the sweet potato slices are cooked, remove them from the oven and let cool slightly.

7. Spread mashed avocado on top of the sweet potato slices.

8. Top with chopped fresh herbs, hemp seeds or chopped nuts (optional), and additional seasoning to taste.

Nutritional value per serving (estimated):

Calories: 350 *Fiber: 8g*
Carbs: 40g *Protein: 4g*
Cholesterol: 0mg *Sodium: 60mg*
Total Fat: 15g

Notes:

- You can use a fork to mash the avocado or blend it in a food processor for a smoother consistency.

- Feel free to experiment with different toppings for your sweet potato toast, such as salsa, roasted vegetables, or a drizzle of balsamic glaze.

- Leftover roasted sweet potato slices can be stored in an airtight container in the refrigerator for up to 3 days and reheated in the oven or microwave.

Sprouted Lentil Breakfast Bowl

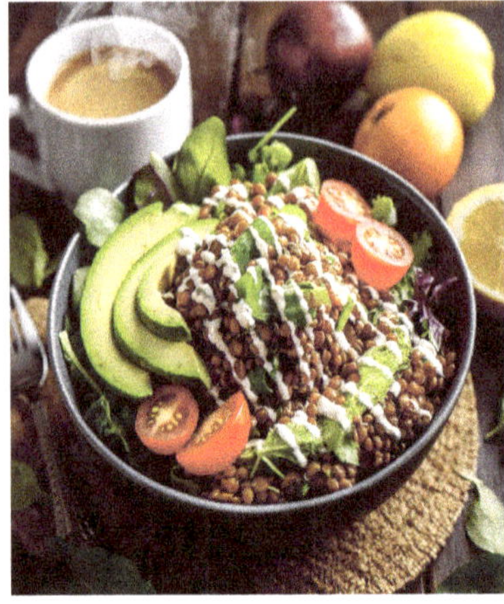

Preparation time: 10 minutes
Cooking time: 20-25 minutes
Servings: 2

Ingredients:
- 1/2 cup sprouted lentils, rinsed and well-drained
- 1/2 cup chopped vegetables (low-FODMAP options like cherry tomatoes, cucumber, bell peppers)
- 1/4 cup chopped fresh herbs, such as parsley, cilantro
- 1 tablespoon olive oil
- 1 tablespoon lemon juice
- Salt and pepper to taste
- Optional toppings: Chopped nuts or seeds, avocado slices, hot sauce

Directions:

1. If you don't have sprouted lentils, you can sprout your own dry brown lentils by soaking them in water for 24-48 hours, rinsing them every 12 hours.
2. Cook the sprouted lentils according to package instructions or until tender.
3. While the lentils are cooking, chop the vegetables and fresh herbs.
4. In a bowl, combine cooked lentils, chopped vegetables, and fresh herbs.
5. In a separate small bowl, whisk together olive oil, lemon juice, salt, and pepper.
6. Pour the dressing over the lentil and vegetable mixture in the bowl.
7. Toss gently to coat.
8. Serve immediately, topped with chopped nuts or seeds, avocado slices, and hot sauce (optional).

Nutritional value per serving (estimated):

Calories: 300

Carbs: 40g

Cholesterol: 0mg

Total Fat: 10g

Fiber: 10g

Protein: 15g

Sodium: 60mg

Notes:

- Sprouting lentils increases their digestibility and nutrient content. However, if you cannot tolerate sprouted lentils, you can use cooked brown lentils instead. Just be mindful of portion sizes, as brown lentils are higher in FODMAPs than sprouted lentils.

- This breakfast bowl is a great source of protein and fiber to keep you feeling full throughout the morning.

- You may customize the toppings to your liking.

Chapter 4: Lunch Recipes

Vegetable Curry with Quinoa

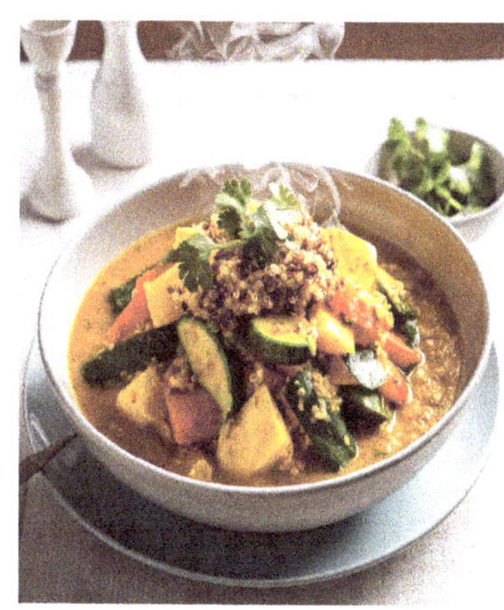

Preparation time: 15 minutes
Cooking time: 25-30 minutes
Servings: 4

Ingredients:

- 1 tablespoon olive oil
- 1 teaspoon curry powder (choose a low-FODMAP option)
- 1/2 teaspoon turmeric
- 1/4 teaspoon ground ginger
- 1 (14.5 oz) can undrained, diced tomatoes
- 1 (15 oz) can chickpeas, drained and rinsed
- 1 cup vegetable broth (low-FODMAP option)
- 1 cup chopped vegetables (low-FODMAP options like carrots, bell peppers, zucchini)
- 1 cup cooked quinoa
- Salt and pepper to taste
- Chopped fresh cilantro (optional)

Directions:
1. Warm olive oil in a large pot or Dutch oven over medium heat.
2. Add curry powder, turmeric, and ground ginger. Continue cooking for an additional minute, stirring constantly, to fully release the aroma of the spices.
3. Pour in the diced tomatoes with their juices and scrape up any browned bits from the bottom of the pot.
4. Add drained and rinsed chickpeas, vegetable broth, and chopped vegetables.
5. Bring the mixture to a boil, then lower the heat and let it simmer for 15-20 minutes, or until the vegetables become tender.
6. Stir in cooked quinoa and heat through for another 2-3 minutes.
7. Season with salt and pepper to taste.
8. Garnish with chopped fresh cilantro (optional) and serve over rice or with gluten-free flatbreads.

Nutritional value per serving (estimated):

Calories: 400

Carbs: 60g

Cholesterol: 0mg

Total Fat: 10g

Fiber: 10g

Protein: 15g

Sodium: 350mg

Notes:

- You can adjust the amount of curry powder to your spice preference.
- Feel free to experiment with different low-FODMAP vegetables in your curry.
- Leftovers can be stored in an airtight container in the refrigerator for up to 3 days and reheated on the stovetop.

Lentil Soup

Preparation time: 15 minutes
Cooking time: 30-35 minutes
Servings: 4-6

Ingredients:
- 1 tablespoon olive oil
- 2 carrots, chopped
- 1 teaspoon dried thyme
- 1/2 teaspoon ground cumin
- 1 cup brown lentils, rinsed
- 4 cups vegetable broth (low-FODMAP option)
- 1 (14.5 oz) can diced, undrained tomatoes
- Salt and pepper to taste
- Chopped fresh parsley (optional)

Directions:
1. Warm olive oil in a large pot or Dutch oven over medium heat. Add the chopped carrot and let it cook until softened, about 5 minutes.
2. Add thyme and cumin. Continue cooking for an additional minute, stirring constantly, to fully release the aroma of the spices.
3. Stir in rinsed brown lentils, vegetable broth, and diced tomatoes with their juices.

4. Bring to a boil, then reduce heat and simmer for 30-35 minutes, or until the lentils are tender.

5. Season with salt and pepper to taste.

6. Garnish with chopped fresh parsley (optional) and serve with a side of crusty bread.

Nutritional value per serving (estimated):

Calories: 300
Carbs: 40g
Cholesterol: 0mg
Total Fat: 5g

Fiber: 15g
Protein: 10g
Sodium: 300mg

Notes:

- You can add other low-FODMAP vegetables to this soup, such as chopped zucchini or green beans.

- If you prefer a smoother soup, you can blend a portion of the cooked soup with an immersion blender.

- Leftovers can be stored in an airtight container in the refrigerator for up to 3 days and reheated on the stovetop.

Coconut Curry Noodle Bowl

***Preparation time: 10 minutes | Cooking time:
10-15 minutes | Servings: 2***

Ingredients:
- 1 tablespoon olive oil
- 1 tablespoon curry powder (choose a low-FODMAP option)
- 1/2 teaspoon turmeric
- 1 (13.5 oz) can light coconut milk
- 1/2 cup vegetable broth (low-FODMAP option)
- 1 cup chopped vegetables (low-FODMAP options like bell peppers, zucchini, carrots)
- 8 oz rice noodles or other low-FODMAP noodles (cooked according to package instructions)
- Salt and pepper to taste
- Chopped fresh cilantro or basil (optional)
- Lime wedges (optional)

Directions:
1. Heat olive oil in a large pan or wok over medium heat.
2. Add curry powder. Continue cooking for an additional minute, stirring constantly, to fully release the aroma of the spices.
3. Stir in turmeric, coconut milk, and vegetable broth.
4. Bring the mixture to a simmer and let it cook for 5 minutes.

5. Add chopped vegetables and cook for another 5-7 minutes, or until tender-crisp.
6. While the vegetables are cooking, cook the rice noodles according to package instructions.
7. Drain the noodles and add them to the pan with the curry sauce.
8. Toss to coat the noodles in the sauce.
9. Season with salt and pepper to taste.
10. Divide the curry and noodles between two bowls.
11. Garnish with chopped fresh cilantro or basil (optional) and lime wedges (optional).

Nutritional value per serving (estimated):

Calories: 400   *Fiber: 5g*
Carbs: 50g   *Protein: 10g*
Cholesterol: 0mg   *Sodium: 250mg*
Total Fat: 15g

Notes:
- You can adjust the amount of curry powder to your spice preference.
- Feel free to experiment with different low-FODMAP vegetables in your curry.
- If you find the curry too thick, you can add a splash more vegetable broth to thin it out.

Stuffed Portobello Mushrooms

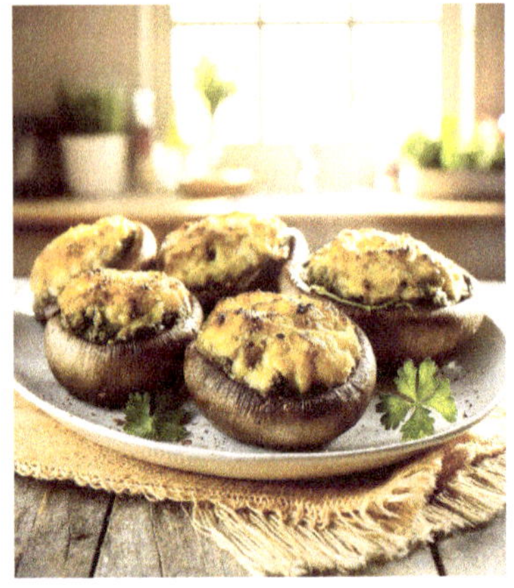

Preparation time: 15 minutes
Cooking time: 20-25 minutes
Servings: 2

Ingredients:
- 2 large portobello mushrooms, stems removed
- 1 tablespoon olive oil
- 1/2 cup chopped vegetables (low-FODMAP options like zucchini, bell peppers, spinach)
- 1/4 cup cooked quinoa (optional)
- 1/4 cup crumbled vegan cheese (choose a low-FODMAP option)
- 1/4 cup chopped fresh herbs (parsley, thyme)
- Salt and pepper to taste

Directions:
1. Preheat oven to 400°F (200°C). Place parchment paper on a baking sheet.

2. Gently wipe clean the portobello mushroom caps with a damp paper towel.

3. Using a spoon, carefully scrape out some of the gills from the underside of the caps to create a well.

4. Brush the tops and insides of the mushroom caps with olive oil.

5. In a pan, heat olive oil over medium heat.

6. Add chopped vegetables. Cook for another 5 minutes, or until the vegetables are softened.

7. Stir in cooked quinoa (if using), crumbled vegan cheese, and chopped fresh herbs. Season with salt and pepper to taste.

8. Spoon the filling mixture evenly into the prepared portobello mushroom caps.

9. Place the stuffed portobello mushrooms on the prepared baking sheet.

10. Bake for 20-25 minutes, or until the mushrooms are tender and the filling is heated through.

11. Broil for the last minute or two to brown the tops of the mushrooms (optional).

12. Serve hot.

Nutritional value per serving (estimated):

Calories: 350

Carbs: 35g

Cholesterol: 0mg

Total Fat: 10g

Fiber: 5g

Protein: 15g

Sodium: 300mg

Notes:

- You can stuff the portobello mushrooms with other low-FODMAP ingredients, such as cooked lentils, crumbled tempeh, or chopped nuts.

- If you don't have vegan cheese, you can omit it or use a sprinkle of nutritional yeast for added flavor.

- Portobello mushrooms are a good source of vitamins and minerals, including potassium, vitamin D, and B vitamins.

Rainbow Veggie Wraps

Preparation time: 10 minutes
Cooking time: N/A
Servings: 4

Ingredients:
- 4 large lettuce leaves or whole wheat tortillas
- 1 cup hummus (choose a low-FODMAP option)
- 1 cup chopped vegetables (various colors for a rainbow effect - choose low-FODMAP options like bell peppers, shredded carrots, cucumber, spinach)
- 1/2 cup cooked chickpeas (optional)
- 1/4 cup crumbled feta cheese (optional - choose a low-FODMAP option)
- Fresh herbs (optional: chopped parsley, cilantro)

Directions:
1. Spread hummus evenly on each tortilla or lettuce leaf.
2. Layer the chopped vegetables in rows or any design you prefer.
3. Add cooked chickpeas (if using) for extra protein and texture.
4. Crumble feta cheese over the top (if using).
5. Garnish with fresh herbs (optional).

6. Roll up the tortillas or fold the lettuce leaves to enclose the filling.

7. Cut the wraps in half diagonally (optional) for easier handling.

8. Serve immediately.

Nutritional value per serving (estimated):

Calories: 350
Carbs: 40g
Cholesterol: 30mg
Total Fat: 15g

Fiber: 10g
Protein: 10g
Sodium: 300mg

Notes:

- You can customize the vegetables in your wraps based on your preferences and what's in season.

- To make vegan wraps, omit the feta cheese and choose a vegan hummus option.

- These wraps are a great and portable lunch option.

Edamame Salad with Quinoa

Preparation time: 10 minutes
Cooking time: 15 minutes (for quinoa)
Servings: 2

Ingredients:
- 1 cup cooked quinoa
- 1 cup shelled edamame, cooked or frozen and thawed
- 1/2 cup chopped vegetables (low-FODMAP options like cucumber, bell peppers, cherry tomatoes)
- 1 tablespoon olive oil
- 1 tablespoon rice vinegar
- 1 teaspoon sesame oil
- 1/2 teaspoon grated ginger (optional)
- Salt and pepper to taste
- Chopped fresh herbs (optional: cilantro, scallions)

Directions:
1. Cook the quinoa according to package instructions if not already cooked.
2. In a bowl, combine cooked quinoa, shelled edamame, and chopped vegetables.

3. In a separate small bowl, whisk together olive oil, rice vinegar, sesame oil, and grated ginger (if using).

4. Pour the dressing over the quinoa, edamame, and vegetable mixture.

5. Toss gently to coat.

6. Season with salt and pepper to taste.

7. Garnish with chopped fresh herbs (optional) and serve chilled or at room temperature.

Nutritional value per serving (estimated):

Calories: 300   *Fiber: 8g*
Carbs: 40g   *Protein: 15g*
Cholesterol: 0mg   *Sodium: 150mg*
Total Fat: 10g

Notes:

- You can add a pinch of red pepper flakes to the dressing for a bit of spice.

- Feel free to experiment with other low-FODMAP chopped vegetables in your salad.

- You can store leftovers in an airtight container in the refrigerator for up to 3 days.

Vegetable Skewers with Tahini Dip

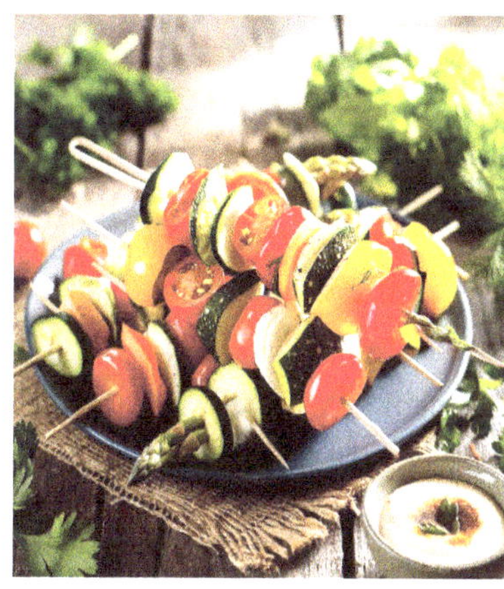

Preparation time: 15 minutes
Cooking time: 10-15 minutes (depending on grilling method)
Servings: 2-3

Ingredients:
For the Skewers:
- Wooden skewers soaked in water for at least 10 minutes (to prevent burning)
- 1 bell pepper, cut into chunks
- 1 zucchini, cut into chunks
- 1 cup cherry tomatoes
- 1 tablespoon olive oil
- Salt and pepper to taste

For the Tahini Dip:
- 1/4 cup tahini
- 1/4 cup lemon juice
- 2 tablespoons water

- 1 tablespoon olive oil
- Salt and pepper to taste

Directions:
1. Preheat oven to broil or prepare your grill for medium heat.
2. Thread the bell pepper chunks, zucchini chunks, and cherry tomatoes onto the soaked wooden skewers, alternating colors for a visually appealing presentation.
3. Brush the skewers with olive oil and season with salt and pepper to taste.
4. Broil the skewers in the preheated oven for 10-12 minutes, or grill for 5-7 minutes per side, until the vegetables are tender-crisp and slightly charred.

For the Tahini Dip:
1. In a small bowl, whisk together tahini, lemon juice, water, and olive oil.
2. Season with salt and pepper to taste.
3. Add a splash more water if the dip is too thick.

Assembly:
1. Serve the grilled vegetable skewers with the tahini dip on the side.

Nutritional value per serving (estimated):

Calories: 300
Carbs: 30g
Cholesterol: 0mg
Total Fat: 15g

Fiber: 5g
Protein: 5g
Sodium: 150mg

Notes:

- You can use other low-FODMAP vegetables for the skewers, such as mushrooms, eggplant, or asparagus.

- If you don't have a grill or broiler, you can cook the vegetables in a pan on the stovetop over medium heat until tender-crisp.

- The tahini dip can be made ahead of time and stored in an airtight container in the refrigerator for up to 3 days.

Quinoa Buddha Bowl

Preparation time: 15 minutes
Cooking time: 15 minutes (for quinoa)
Servings: 2

Ingredients:
- 1 cup cooked quinoa
- 1/2 cup chopped vegetables (low-FODMAP options like shredded carrots, bell peppers, cucumber)
- 1/4 cup cooked chickpeas
- 1/4 cup baked tempeh (optional)
- 1 tablespoon olive oil
- 1 tablespoon lemon juice
- 1/2 teaspoon dried herbs (Italian seasoning, thyme)
- Salt and pepper to taste
- Chopped fresh herbs (optional: parsley, cilantro)
- Avocado slices (optional)

Directions:
1. Cook the quinoa according to package instructions if not already cooked.
2. In a large bowl, combine cooked quinoa, chopped vegetables, and cooked chickpeas (and tempeh, if using).

3. In a separate small bowl, whisk together olive oil, lemon juice, dried herbs, salt, and pepper.
4. Pour the dressing over the quinoa and vegetable mixture in the bowl.
5. Toss gently to coat.
6. Garnish with chopped fresh herbs (optional) and avocado slices (optional).

Nutritional value per serving (estimated):

Calories: 400   *Fiber: 10g*
Carbs: 50g   *Protein: 20g*
Cholesterol: 50mg   *Sodium: 200mg*
Total Fat: 15g

Notes:

- You can customize the vegetables and protein in your Buddha bowl based on your preferences and what's in season.

- This is a complete and balanced meal that is perfect for lunch or dinner.

- You can store leftovers in an airtight container in the refrigerator for up to 3 days.

Lentil and Vegetable Burgers

Preparation time: 15 minutes | Cooking time: 20-25 minutes | Servings: 2-3

Ingredients:
- 1 cup cooked brown lentils
- 1/2 cup chopped vegetables (low-FODMAP options like zucchini, bell peppers, mushrooms)
- 1/4 cup rolled oats
- 1/4 cup chopped fresh herbs e.g parsley, cilantro
- 1 tablespoon olive oil
- 1 tablespoon lemon juice
- 1/2 teaspoon ground cumin
- Salt and pepper to taste
- Gluten-free buns (toasted, optional)
- Low-FODMAP burger toppings (e.g., lettuce, tomato)

Directions:
1. In a large bowl, mash the cooked brown lentils with a fork, leaving some texture.
2. Add chopped vegetables, rolled oats, chopped fresh herbs, olive oil, lemon juice, cumin, salt, and pepper.
3. Mix well to combine and form a thick patty mixture. If the mixture feels too loose, add a tablespoon more of rolled oats.

4. Shape the lentil mixture into two or three equal burger patties.

5. Heat a pan or grill over medium heat. Apply a light coat of olive oil using a brush or spray.

6. Cook the lentil burgers for 5-7 minutes per side, or until browned and cooked through.

7. Toast gluten-free buns (optional) and assemble your burgers with your favorite low-FODMAP toppings.

Nutritional value per serving (estimated):

Calories: 350
Carbs: 40g
Cholesterol: 0mg
Total Fat: 10g

Fiber: 10g
Protein: 15g
Sodium: 250mg

Notes:

- You can experiment with different low-FODMAP vegetables in your lentil burgers.

- If you don't have rolled oats, you can use another gluten-free flour option like almond flour or oat flour.

- Leftover lentil burgers can be stored in an airtight container in the refrigerator for up to 3 days and reheated in a pan or microwave.

Coconut Curry Chickpea Salad Sandwich

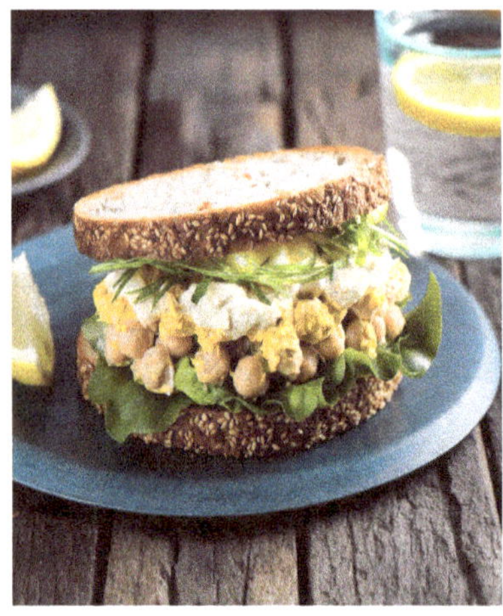

Preparation time: 10 minutes
Cooking time: N/A (depending on chickpeas)
Servings: 1

Ingredients:
- 2 slices gluten-free bread
- 1/2 cup cooked chickpeas
- 1/4 cup chopped vegetables (low-FODMAP options like bell peppers, cucumber)
- 2 tablespoons chopped fresh herbs such as cilantro, parsley
- 1 tablespoon light coconut milk
- 1 teaspoon curry powder (low-FODMAP option)
- 1/4 teaspoon lime juice
- Salt and pepper to taste

Directions:

1. If using dried chickpeas, cook them according to package instructions or until tender. You can also use canned chickpeas, drained and rinsed.

2. In a bowl, mash about half of the chickpeas with a fork for a chunky texture. Leave the other half whole.

3. Add chopped vegetables, chopped fresh herbs, light coconut milk, curry powder, lime juice, salt, and pepper.

4. Gently mix to combine all ingredients.

5. Toast your gluten-free bread slices (optional).

6. Spread the chickpea salad mixture on one slice of bread.

7. Place the other slice of bread on top and savor your creation!

Nutritional value per serving (estimated):

Calories: 350
Carbs: 45g
Cholesterol: 0mg
Total Fat: 10g

Fiber: 5g
Protein: 10g
Sodium: 200mg

Notes:

- You can adjust the amount of curry powder to your spice preference.

- Feel free to experiment with other chopped low-FODMAP vegetables in your salad, such as shredded carrots or chopped celery.
- This is a quick and easy vegetarian lunch option that is packed with protein and fiber.

Chapter 5: Dinner Recipes

Stir-Fried Noodles with Tofu

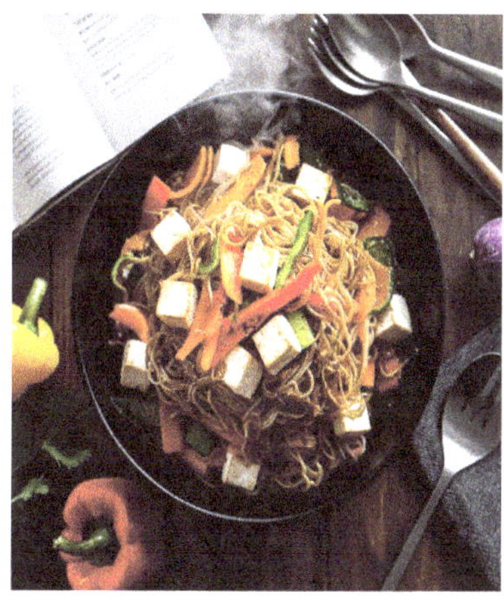

Preparation time: 10 minutes
Cooking time: 15-20 minutes
Servings: 2

Ingredients:

- 8 oz rice noodles or other low-FODMAP noodles (e.g., mung bean noodles, buckwheat noodles) - cooked according to package instructions

- 1 block extra firm, low-FODMAP tofu, drained and pressed

- 1 tablespoon low-FODMAP oil (e.g., avocado oil, grapeseed oil)

- 1/2 cup chopped low-FODMAP vegetables (e.g., carrots, green beans, snow peas)

- 1 tablespoon low-FODMAP soy sauce (tamari)

- 1 tablespoon rice vinegar

- 1/2 teaspoon grated ginger (optional)

- Salt and black pepper to taste
- Chopped fresh herbs (optional: cilantro, Thai basil) - for garnish

Directions:

1. Wrap the drained tofu block in a clean kitchen towel or paper towels. Place a heavy object (like a cast iron skillet or a pot filled with water) on top to press out excess moisture for at least 15 minutes.

2. While the tofu presses, cook the rice noodles or other low-FODMAP noodles according to package instructions. After cooking, drain the ingredients and rinse them with cold water to prevent sticking. Set aside.

3. Once pressed, cut the tofu into bite-sized cubes. Warm the oil in a large pan or wok over medium-high heat. Add the tofu cubes and cook for 5-7 minutes per side, or until golden brown and slightly crispy. Move the cooked tofu to a plate.

4. In the same pan, add the chopped low-FODMAP vegetables. Cook for 3-4 minutes, or until tender-crisp.

5. In a small bowl, whisk together the low-FODMAP soy sauce, rice vinegar, and grated ginger (if using). Add the sauce to the pan with the vegetables and mix everything together. Add the cooked noodles and cooked tofu back to the pan.

6. Toss everything together gently to coat the noodles and tofu in the sauce. Season with salt and black pepper to taste.

7. Divide the stir-fried noodles with tofu between two plates and garnish with chopped fresh herbs (optional). Enjoy immediately.

Nutritional value per serving (estimated):

Calories: 400

Carbs: 50g

Cholesterol: 0mg

Total Fat: 15g

Fiber: 5g

Protein: 20g

Sodium: 350mg

Notes:

- You can adjust the amount of low-FODMAP soy sauce to your taste preference.

- Feel free to experiment with other low-FODMAP vegetables in your stir-fry, such as shredded bell peppers or chopped mushrooms.

- This is a quick and easy vegan meal that is packed with protein and fiber.

Thai Green Curry with Vegetables

Preparation time: 15 minutes | Cooking time: 20-25 minutes | Servings: 2

Ingredients:
- 1 tablespoon low-FODMAP oil (e.g., avocado oil, grapeseed oil)
- 1 green bell pepper, sliced
- 1 zucchini, sliced
- 1 cup broccoli florets
- 1 can (13.5 oz) coconut milk (choose a low-FODMAP brand)
- 1 tablespoon green curry paste (low-FODMAP option)
- 1 tablespoon lime juice
- 1/2 cup vegetable broth (low-FODMAP option)
- 1/4 cup chopped green beans
- 1 tablespoon rice vinegar
- 1 tablespoon chopped fresh cilantro
- Salt and black pepper to taste
- Cooked rice (optional)

Directions:
1. Warm the oil in a large pot or Dutch oven over medium heat. Add the sliced green bell pepper, zucchini, and broccoli florets. Cook for 5-7 minutes, or until tender-crisp.
2. Stir in the green curry paste and cook for another minute, stirring constantly, to release the fragrant flavors.

3. Pour in the coconut milk, vegetable broth, and lime juice. Bring the mixture to a simmer and let it cook for 5 minutes.

4. Add the chopped green beans and rice vinegar. Simmer for another 5-7 minutes, or until the green beans are tender-crisp and the vegetables are cooked through.

5. Add salt and black pepper according to your taste preferences.

6. Stir in the chopped fresh cilantro just before serving.

7. Serve the Thai green curry with vegetables over cooked rice (optional).

Nutritional value per serving (estimated):

- Calories: 350
- Carbs: 40g
- Cholesterol: 0mg
- Total Fat: 15g

- Fiber: 10g
- Protein: 5g
- Sodium: 150mg

Notes:

- You can adjust the amount of green curry paste to your spice preference.

- Feel free to experiment with other low-FODMAP vegetables in your curry, such as sliced carrots, chopped snow peas, or baby corn.

Vegan Chili

Preparation time: 15 minutes
Cooking time: 30-35 minutes
Servings: 4-6

Ingredients:
- 1 tablespoon olive oil
- 2 carrots, chopped
- 1 teaspoon ground cumin
- 1 teaspoon chili powder (low-FODMAP option)
- 1/2 teaspoon smoked paprika
- 1 (15 oz) can diced, undrained tomatoes
- 1 (15 oz) can kidney beans, drained and rinsed (choose low-FODMAP option)
- 1 (15 oz) can black beans, drained and rinsed
- 4 cups vegetable broth (low-FODMAP option)
- 1 cup chopped green bell pepper
- 1/2 cup chopped zucchini
- Salt and black pepper to taste
- Chopped fresh cilantro (optional)
- Vegan sour cream (optional) - for garnish
- Avocado slices (optional) - for garnish

Directions:

1. Heat the olive oil in a large pot or Dutch oven over medium heat. Add the chopped carrots. Let it cook for 5 minutes, or until softened.

2. Add cumin, chili powder, and smoked paprika. Let the mixture cook for an additional minute, stirring constantly, to release the aroma of the spices.

3. Add the diced tomatoes along with their juices. Use a spatula to scrape up any browned bits from the bottom of the pot.

4. Stir in the drained and rinsed kidney beans and black beans.

5. Add the vegetable broth and bring to a boil. Then, reduce heat and simmer for 20-25 minutes, or until the vegetables are tender and the chili has thickened slightly.

6. While the chili simmers, chop the green bell pepper and zucchini.

7. After 20-25 minutes of simmering, add the chopped green pepper and zucchini to the pot. Simmer for another 5-7 minutes, or until the vegetables are tender-crisp.

8. Season with salt and black pepper according to your taste preferences.

9. Taste and adjust the seasonings as needed. You can add a pinch of red pepper flakes for extra spice (optional).

10. Serve the vegan chili hot in bowls. Garnish with chopped fresh cilantro. Vegan sour cream and avocado slices also make delicious toppings (optional).

Nutritional value per serving (estimated):

- Calories: 350
- Carbs: 50g
- Cholesterol: 0mg
- Total Fat: 10g

- Fiber: 15g
- Protein: 15g
- Sodium: 300mg

Notes:

- You can add other low-FODMAP vegetables to this chili, such as chopped mushrooms or chopped corn. To avoid high-FODMAP onions, you can use green onions instead.

- If you prefer a smoother chili, you can use an immersion blender to blend a portion of the cooked chili.

- Leftovers can be stored in an airtight container in the refrigerator for up to 3 days and reheated on the stovetop.

Stuffed Sweet Potatoes

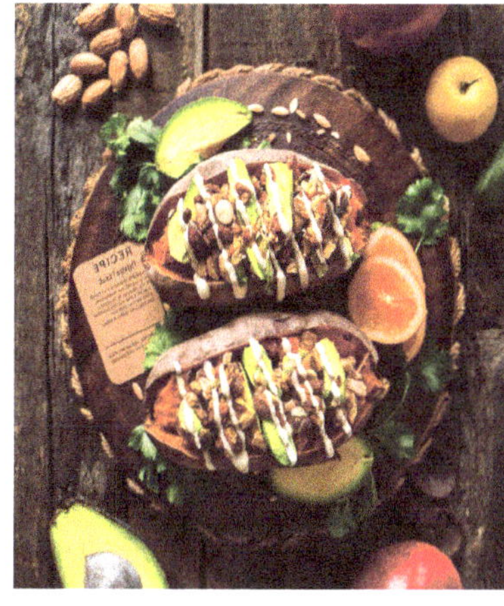

Preparation time: 15 minutes
Cooking time: 45-50 minutes
Servings: 2

Ingredients:
- 2 medium sweet potatoes
- 1 tablespoon olive oil
- 1 cup chopped bell peppers (red, yellow, or orange
- choose a low-FODMAP option)
  1 zucchini, chopped
- 1/2 cup cooked black beans, rinsed and drained (choose low-FODMAP option)
- 1/4 cup chopped fresh herbs e.g parsley, cilantro
- 1/4 cup chopped walnuts or pecans (optional)
- 1 tablespoon low-FODMAP tomato paste
- 1/4 cup vegetable broth (low-FODMAP option)
- Salt and black pepper to taste
- Chopped fresh herbs (optional) - for garnish

Directions:

1. Preheat oven to 400°F (200°C). Wash the sweet potatoes and pierce the skin with a fork a few times.

2. Place the sweet potatoes on a baking sheet and roast for 45-50 minutes, or until tender when pierced through with a fork.

3. While the sweet potatoes roast, heat the olive oil in a large skillet over medium heat. Add the bell peppers. Cook for about 5 minutes or until the ingredients have softened.

4. Add the chopped zucchini and cook for another 2-3 minutes, or until the zucchini is tender-crisp.

5. Stir in the cooked black beans, chopped fresh herbs, and chopped walnuts or pecans (if using).

6. Add the low-FODMAP tomato paste and vegetable broth to the pan. Use a spatula to scrape up any browned bits from the bottom of the skillet.

7. Season with salt and black pepper to taste. Bring to a simmer and cook for 5 minutes, or until the mixture thickens slightly.

8. Once the sweet potatoes are cooked, remove them from the oven and let them cool slightly for a few minutes.

9. Slice the sweet potatoes open lengthwise and carefully fluff up the flesh with a fork.

10. Spoon the prepared vegetable and bean mixture evenly into the hollowed-out sweet potatoes.

11. Garnish with additional chopped fresh herbs (optional) and serve hot.

Nutritional value per serving (estimated):

- Calories: 450	*- Fiber: 10g*
- Carbs: 60g	*- Protein: 10g*
- Cholesterol: 0mg	*- Sodium: 200mg*
- Total Fat: 15g	

Notes:

- You can experiment with other low-FODMAP vegetables in your stuffing, such as chopped mushrooms or chopped green beans.

- If you don't have walnuts or pecans, you can omit them or use another low-FODMAP nut option like chopped almonds.

- Stuffed sweet potatoes are a delicious and nutritious vegan meal that is perfect for lunch or dinner.

Lentil Shepherd's Pie

Preparation time: 15 minutes
Cooking time: 40-45 minutes
Servings: 4

Ingredients:
- 1 tablespoon olive oil
- 2 carrots, chopped
- 1 teaspoon dried thyme
- 1/2 teaspoon dried rosemary
- 1 cup cooked brown lentils
- 1 (15 oz) can diced, undrained tomatoes
- 1 1/2 cups vegetable broth (low-FODMAP option)
- Salt and black pepper to taste
- 1 tablespoon cornstarch (optional)
- 2 cups mashed potatoes (made with low-FODMAP potatoes like russet or Yukon gold)

Directions:
1. Preheat oven to 400°F (200°C).
2. Warm the olive oil in a large pot or Dutch oven over medium heat. Add the carrots and let them cook for 5 minutes, or until it becomes tender.

3. Add the dried thyme, and dried rosemary. Let the mixture cook for an additional minute, stirring it constantly, to release the aroma of the herbs.

4. Stir in the cooked brown lentils and diced tomatoes with their juices.

5. Add the vegetable broth and gently bring to a simmer. Reduce heat and cook for 20-25 minutes, or until the vegetables are tender and the lentils are heated through.

6. Add salt and black pepper to your desired taste. **Thicken the sauce (optional):** If you prefer a thicker filling, whisk together 1 tablespoon cornstarch with a little cold water to make a slurry. Stir the slurry into the simmering lentil mixture and cook for an additional minute or two, until the sauce thickens slightly.

7. While the lentil mixture simmers, prepare your mashed potatoes using low-FODMAP potatoes like russet or Yukon gold. Be sure to avoid using high-FODMAP ingredients like milk or cream cheese. Season the mashed potatoes with salt and pepper to taste.

8. Transfer the lentil mixture to a baking dish or casserole dish. Spread the mashed potatoes evenly over the top, creating a smooth layer.

9. Bake in the preheated oven for 15-20 minutes, or until the mashed potatoes are golden brown and heated through.

10. Let the shepherd's pie cool slightly before serving. Enjoy hot!

Nutritional value per serving (estimated):

- *Calories: 400*
- *Carbs: 55g*
- *Cholesterol: 0mg*
- *Total Fat: 10g*

- *Fiber: 15g*
- *Protein: 20g*
- *Sodium: 300mg*

Notes:

- You can experiment with other low-FODMAP vegetables in your lentil filling, such as chopped mushrooms or chopped green beans.

- You can store leftovers in an airtight container in the refrigerator for up to 3 days. Reheat them in the oven or microwave when ready to enjoy again.

Coconut Curry Lentil Soup

Preparation time: 15 minutes | Cooking time: 30-35 minutes | Servings: 4

Ingredients:
- 1 tablespoon olive oil
- 2 carrots, chopped
- 1 tablespoon curry powder (low-FODMAP option)
- 1 teaspoon ground ginger
- 1 (14 oz) can diced tomatoes, undrained
- 1 (15 oz) can cooked lentils, rinsed and drained
- 4 cups vegetable broth (low-FODMAP option)
- 1 cup light coconut milk (choose a low-FODMAP brand)
- Salt and black pepper to taste
- Chopped fresh cilantro (optional) - for garnish
- Lime wedges (optional) - for garnish

Directions:
1. Heat the olive oil in a large pot or Dutch oven over medium heat. Add the chopped carrots and let them cook until softened, approximately 5 minutes.
2. Add curry powder and ground ginger. Stir constantly and cook for another minute to release the spices' aroma.
3. Pour diced tomatoes with their juices into the pot, scraping up any browned bits from the bottom.
4. Stir in the rinsed and drained lentils, vegetable broth, and light coconut milk.

5. Bring to a boil, then reduce heat and simmer for 20-25 minutes, or until the vegetables are tender and the soup has thickened slightly.

6. Add salt and black pepper according to your taste preference. You can adjust the amount of curry powder for your desired spice level.

7. Taste and adjust the seasonings as needed.

8. Serve the coconut curry lentil soup hot in bowls. Garnish with chopped fresh cilantro (optional) and lime wedges (optional).

Nutritional value per serving (estimated):

- *Calories: 350*
- *Carbs: 50g*
- *Cholesterol: 0mg*
- *Total Fat: 10g*

- *Fiber: 15g*
- *Protein: 15g*
- *Sodium: 300mg*

Notes:

- You can add other low-FODMAP vegetables to this soup, such as chopped green beans or chopped mushrooms.

- To make the soup creamier, you can use an immersion blender to blend a portion of the cooked soup.

- Leftovers can be stored in an airtight container in the refrigerator for up to 3 days and reheated on the stovetop.

Vegan Paella

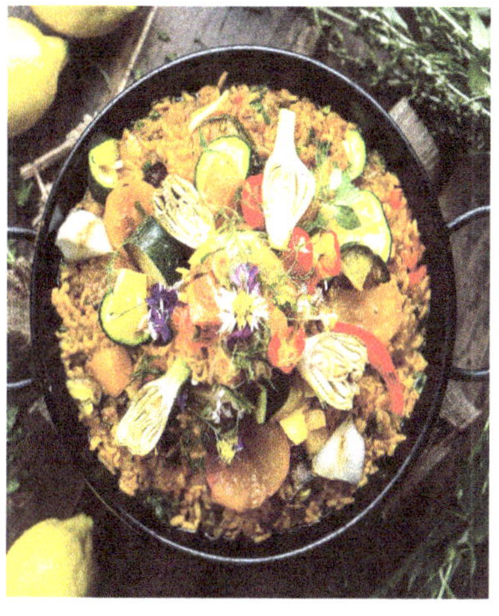

Preparation time: 15 minutes
Cooking time: 30-35 minutes
Servings: 4

Ingredients:
- 1 tablespoon olive oil
- 1 bell pepper (red, yellow, or orange - choose a low-FODMAP option) chopped
- 1 zucchini, chopped
- 1 cup chopped low-FODMAP tomatoes (e.g., peeled tomatoes, chopped cherry tomatoes)
- 1 cup vegetable broth (low-FODMAP option)
- 1 1/2 cups cooked artichoke hearts, quartered (look for low-FODMAP canned artichokes)
- 1 cup cooked green peas (fresh or frozen)
- 1 cup short-grain rice (rinsed)
- 1/2 teaspoon smoked paprika
- 1/4 teaspoon saffron threads (optional)

- Salt and black pepper to taste

- Chopped fresh parsley (optional) - for garnish

Directions:

1. Heat the olive oil in a large pan or paella pan (if you have one) over medium heat. Add the chopped bell pepper, allowing it to cook for about 5 minutes, or until softened.

2. Add the chopped zucchini and cook for another 2-3 minutes, or until the zucchini is tender-crisp.

3. Stir in the chopped low-FODMAP tomatoes and vegetable broth. Let it gently simmer and cook for about 5 minutes.

4. Add the quartered artichoke hearts, cooked green peas, rinsed short-grain rice, smoked paprika, and saffron threads (if using).

5. Add salt and black pepper to your desired taste. Stir everything together gently to combine.

6. Bring the mixture to a boil, then reduce heat to low and cover the pan. Let it simmer for 20-25 minutes or until the rice is fully cooked and the liquid has been absorbed.

7. Once the rice is cooked, remove the pan from the heat and let it sit for 5 minutes with the lid on, allowing the flavors to meld.

8. Fluff the rice with a fork before serving.

9. Garnish with chopped fresh parsley (optional) and enjoy your vegan paella!

Nutritional value per serving (estimated):

Calories: 400
Carbs: 60g
Cholesterol: 0mg
Total Fat: 15g

Fiber: 10g
Protein: 10g
Sodium: 300mg

Notes:

- You can experiment with other low-FODMAP vegetables in your paella, such as chopped mushrooms or chopped asparagus.

- If you don't have saffron threads, you can omit them or use a pinch of ground turmeric for a similar color.

- Leftovers can be stored in an airtight container in the refrigerator for up to 3 days and reheated on the stovetop.

Vegetable Fajitas

*Preparation time: 10 minutes | Cooking time:
15-20 minutes | Servings: 2*

Ingredients:
- 1 tablespoon olive oil
- 1 bell pepper (red, yellow, or orange - choose a low-FODMAP option), sliced
- 1 zucchini, sliced
- 1/2 cup chopped low-FODMAP mushrooms (e.g., white mushrooms, portobello mushrooms)
- 1 tablespoon low-FODMAP taco seasoning (choose a brand suitable for low-FODMAP)
- Salt and black pepper to taste
- Corn tortillas (low-FODMAP option) - warmed
- Low-FODMAP toppings (e.g., shredded lettuce, chopped avocado, salsa, chopped cilantro) - for serving

Directions:

1. Heat the olive oil in a large skillet or pan over medium-high heat. Add the sliced bell pepper, zucchini, and mushrooms.

2. Cook for 5-7 minutes, or until the vegetables are tender-crisp and slightly browned.

3. Stir in the low-FODMAP taco seasoning and cook for another minute, coating the vegetables evenly.

4. Season with salt and black pepper to taste.

5. Warm your corn tortillas according to package instructions (microwave, stovetop, or toaster oven).

6. Serve the fajita vegetables on warmed tortillas. Let everyone customize their fajitas with their favorite low-FODMAP toppings like shredded lettuce, chopped avocado, salsa, and chopped cilantro.

Nutritional value per serving (estimated):

Calories: 350   *Fiber: 10g*
Carbs: 45g   *Protein: 5g*
Cholesterol: 0mg   *Sodium: 300mg*
Total Fat: 15g

Notes:

- You can add other low-FODMAP vegetables to your fajitas, such as sliced green beans or chopped cherry tomatoes.

- If you don't have low-FODMAP taco seasoning, you can create your own by mixing together low-FODMAP spices like chili powder, cumin, paprika, and oregano.

Creamy Tomato Pasta with Tofu Scramble

Preparation time: 15 minutes | Cooking time: 15-20 minutes | Servings: 2

Ingredients:
For the Tofu Scramble:
- 1 block extra firm, low-FODMAP tofu, drained and pressed
- 1/4 cup chopped low-FODMAP mushrooms (e.g., white mushrooms, portobello mushrooms)
- 1/4 cup chopped green bell pepper (red, yellow, or orange - choose a low-FODMAP option)
- 1/4 teaspoon turmeric powder
- 1/4 teaspoon smoked paprika
- Salt and black pepper to taste
- 1 tablespoon olive oil

For the Creamy Tomato Sauce:
- 1 tablespoon olive oil
- 1/2 cup chopped low-FODMAP tomatoes (e.g., peeled tomatoes, chopped cherry tomatoes)
- 1/4 cup vegetable broth (low-FODMAP option)
- 1/4 cup unsweetened almond milk or coconut milk (choose a low-FODMAP brand)
- 1 tablespoon nutritional yeast (optional)
- Salt and black pepper to taste
- Cooked low-FODMAP pasta (e.g., rice noodles, gluten-free pasta)

Directions:

1. Crumble the drained and pressed tofu using a fork or your hands.

2. Heat the olive oil in a large skillet or pan over medium heat. Add the chopped mushrooms and green pepper. Cook for about 5 minutes, or until the ingredients have softened.

3. Add the crumbled tofu to the pan and cook for another 5 minutes, stirring occasionally, until the tofu is slightly browned and heated through.

4. Stir in the turmeric powder, smoked paprika, salt, and black pepper to the tofu mixture.

5. While the tofu scramble cooks, heat another tablespoon of olive oil in a separate pan over medium heat.

6. Stir in the chopped low-FODMAP tomatoes, vegetable broth, and unsweetened almond milk (or coconut milk). Let it gently simmer and cook for 5 minutes.

7. Using an immersion blender (or transferring the sauce to a blender), blend the creamy tomato sauce until slightly smooth. You can adjust the consistency to your preference - leave it a little chunky or blend it completely smooth.

8. Add salt and black pepper to taste to the sauce. If you're using nutritional yeast for a cheesy flavor, stir it in as well.

9. In the meantime, cook your chosen low-FODMAP pasta according to package instructions. After cooking, drain the pasta and then put it back into the pot.

10. Pour the creamy tomato sauce over the cooked pasta and toss to coat evenly.

11. Gently fold in the prepared tofu scramble with the vegetables.

12. Serve the creamy tomato pasta with tofu scramble hot and enjoy!

Nutritional value per serving (estimated):

Calories: 450

Carbs: 55g

Cholesterol: 0mg

Total Fat: 15g

Fiber: 10g

Protein: 20g

Sodium: 300mg

Notes:

- You can experiment with other low-FODMAP vegetables in your tofu scramble, such as chopped spinach or chopped asparagus.

- If you don't have nutritional yeast, you can omit it or use a sprinkle of vegan parmesan cheese (check for low-FODMAP options).

- Leftovers can be stored in an airtight container in the refrigerator for up to 3 days and reheated on the stovetop.

Coconut Curry Chickpea Bowls

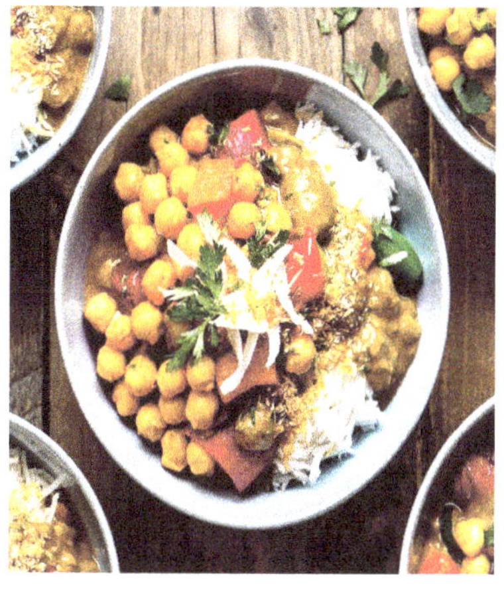

Preparation time: 15 minutes
Cooking time: 20-25 minutes
Servings: 2

Ingredients:
- 1 tablespoon olive oil
- 1 carrot, chopped
- 1 tablespoon curry powder (low-FODMAP option)
- 1 teaspoon ground ginger
- 1 (15 oz) can undrained, diced tomatoes
- 1 (15 oz) can chickpeas, drained and rinsed (choose a low-FODMAP option)
- 1 cup light coconut milk (choose a low-FODMAP brand)
- 1/4 cup vegetable broth (low-FODMAP option)
- Salt and black pepper to taste
- Cooked rice (optional)
- Chopped fresh cilantro (optional) - for garnish
- Lime wedges (optional) - for garnish

Directions:

1. Heat the olive oil in a large pot or Dutch oven over medium heat. Add the chopped carrot, allowing it to cook for 5 minutes, or until softened.

2. Add curry powder and ground ginger. Continue cooking for an additional minute, stirring constantly to release the aroma of the spices.

3. Add the diced tomatoes along with their juices to the pot. Use a spatula to scrape up any browned bits from the bottom of the pot.

4. Stir in the drained and rinsed chickpeas, light coconut milk, and vegetable broth.

5. Bring to a simmer and cook for 15-20 minutes, or until the vegetables are tender and the chickpeas are heated through.

6. Add salt and black pepper according to your taste preference. You can adjust the amount of curry powder for your desired spice level.

7. Taste and adjust the seasonings as needed.

To Assemble the Bowls:

1. Divide the cooked rice (if using) between two bowls.

2. Spoon the coconut curry chickpea mixture over the rice.

3. Garnish with chopped fresh cilantro (optional) and lime wedges (optional).

Nutritional value per serving (estimated):

Calories: 400 *Fiber: 15g*
Carbs: 50g *Protein: 15g*
Cholesterol: 0mg *Sodium: 300mg*
Total Fat: 15g

Notes:

- You can add other low-FODMAP vegetables to your curry, such as chopped green beans or chopped bell peppers.

- To make the curry thicker, you can mash a portion of the chickpeas with a fork before adding them to the pot.

- Leftovers can be stored in an airtight container in the refrigerator for up to 3 days and reheated on the stovetop.

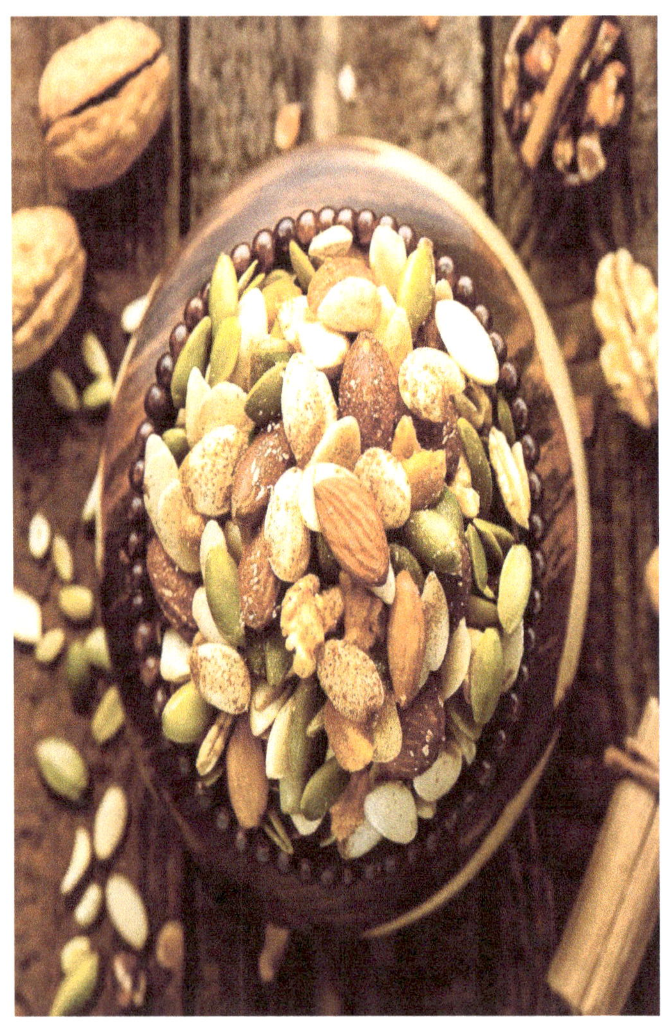

Chapter 6: Dessert/Snack Recipes

Baked Apple with Cinnamon and Walnuts

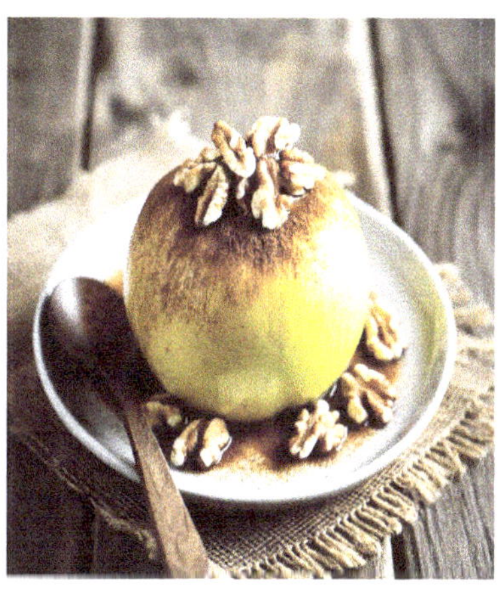

Preparation time: 10 minutes
Cooking time: 30-35 minutes
Servings: 1

Ingredients:

- 1 apple (choose a low-FODMAP variety like Granny Smith or Gala)
- 1 tablespoon ground flaxseed meal
- 3 tablespoons water
- 1/2 teaspoon ground cinnamon
- Pinch of ground nutmeg (optional)
- Chopped walnuts (optional) - limited amount due to high FODMAP content in larger servings

Directions:

1. Preheat oven to 375°F (190°C).

2. Wash the apple and core it from the top, leaving the bottom intact. You can use a spoon or apple corer to create a hollow center.

3. In a small bowl, mix together the ground flaxseed meal and water. Allow the mixture to sit for a few minutes to thicken. This will create a vegan "egg wash."

4. Brush the inside of the apple with the flaxseed mixture.

5. Sprinkle the ground cinnamon and nutmeg (if using) inside the hollowed-out apple.

6. You can add a very small amount of chopped walnuts for a bit of crunch (be mindful of portion size due to FODMAP content in walnuts).

7. Place the stuffed apple in a baking dish and bake for 30-35 minutes, or until the apple is tender when pierced with a fork.

8. Let the baked apple cool slightly before serving. Savor it either warm or at room temperature.

Nutritional value per serving (estimated):

Calories: 150 *Fiber: 5g*
Carbs: 30g *Protein: 1g*
Cholesterol: 0mg *Sodium: 2mg*
Total Fat: 1g

Notes:

- You can experiment with other low-FODMAP spices like ground ginger or cardamom instead of nutmeg.

- If you don't have a ground flaxseed meal, you can use 1 tablespoon of mashed banana as a substitute for the vegan "egg wash."

- For a sweeter option, you can drizzle a small amount of maple syrup over the baked apple before serving (be mindful of portion size due to FODMAP content in maple syrup).

Homemade Rice Cakes with Guacamole

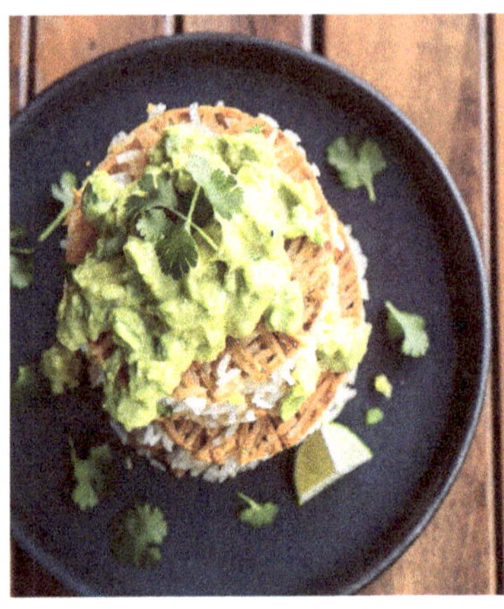

Preparation time: 15 minutes
Cooking time: 20-25 minutes
Servings: 2-3

Ingredients:
For the Rice Cakes:

- 1 cup cooked brown rice (rinsed before cooking)
- 1/4 cup gram flour (also known as chickpea flour)
- 1/4 cup water
- Pinch of salt

For the Guacamole:

- 1 ripe avocado, mashed
- 1 tablespoon chopped red onion (limited amount due to high FODMAP content in larger servings)
- 1 tablespoon lime juice
- Salt and black pepper to taste

Directions:

Prepare the Rice Cakes:

1. In a large bowl, mash the cooked brown rice with a fork or potato masher until mostly broken down but still slightly textured.

2. Stir in the gram flour, water, and salt. Thoroughly combine the ingredients until a thick dough forms.

3. If the dough feels too sticky, add a little more gram flour by tablespoonfuls until it becomes manageable.

4. Divide the dough into 6-8 equal portions. Shape each portion into a small, flat patty.

5. You can cook the rice cakes in a non-stick pan with a light coating of oil over medium heat for 3-4 minutes per side, or until golden brown and crispy. Alternatively, preheat your oven to 375°F (190°C) and bake the rice cakes on a lined baking sheet for 15-20 minutes, flipping them halfway through, until crispy.

Prepare the Guacamole:

1. While the rice cakes cook, mash the ripe avocado in a bowl.

2. Stir in the chopped red onion (limited amount), lime juice, salt, and black pepper to taste.

3. Serve the rice cakes warm with the guacamole for dipping.

Nutritional value per serving (estimated):

Calories: 250	*Fiber: 5g*
Carbs: 35g	*Protein: 5g*
Cholesterol: 0mg	*Sodium: 150mg*
Total Fat: 10g	

Notes:

- You can add a pinch of your favorite low-FODMAP spices like ground cumin to the rice cake dough for extra flavor.

- Leftover rice cakes can be stored in an airtight container at room temperature for up to 2 days or refrigerated for up to 5 days. Reheat them in a pan or toaster oven before serving.

Frozen Banana Bites

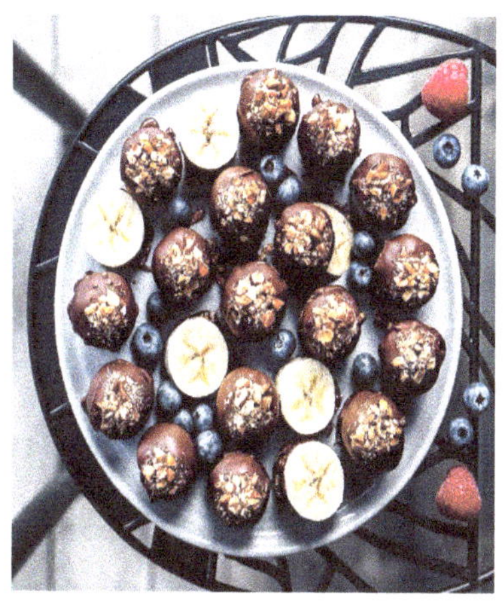

Preparation time: 10 minutes
Freezing time: At least 2 hours, preferably overnight
Servings: 2-3

Ingredients:
- 2 ripe bananas (peeled)

Optional toppings (choose low-FODMAP options):
- Chopped nuts (limited amount due to high FODMAP content in larger servings)
- Shredded unsweetened coconut
- Dried fruit (limited amount due to high FODMAP content in larger servings) like chopped cranberries or blueberries
- Melted dark chocolate (choose a low-FODMAP brand)

Directions:

1. Slice the bananas into bite-sized pieces. You can slice them into rounds, half-moons, or even smaller chunks depending on your preference.

2. Place parchment paper on a baking sheet. Arrange the banana slices in a single layer on the prepared baking sheet, making sure they are not touching.

3. Freeze the banana slices for at least 2 hours, or preferably overnight, until they are frozen solid.

Once frozen, you can enjoy the banana bites plain or customize them with your favorite toppings:

- **With Toppings**: If using toppings, spread a thin layer of melted dark chocolate (optional) over a baking sheet lined with parchment paper. Dip the frozen banana slices into the melted chocolate, coating them completely or partially. Immediately sprinkle with your chosen low-FODMAP toppings (limited amounts of chopped nuts, shredded coconut, or chopped dried fruit). Place the chocolate-dipped banana bites back on the lined baking sheet and freeze for another 15-20 minutes, or until the chocolate is set.

- **Plain**: Enjoy the frozen banana bites plain for a simple and refreshing treat.

Nutritional value per serving (estimated - plain banana bites):

Calories: 100   *Fiber: 3g*
Carbs: 25g   *Protein: 1g*
Cholesterol: 0mg   *Sodium: 1mg*
Total Fat: 0.5g

Notes:

- Frozen banana bites are a healthy and delicious snack that is perfect for satisfying a sweet tooth.

- You can experiment with different low-FODMAP dipping options like melted nut butter (limited amount) or a mixture of mashed berries.

- Leftover frozen banana bites can be stored in an airtight container in the freezer for up to 3 months.

Trail Mix with Nuts and Seeds

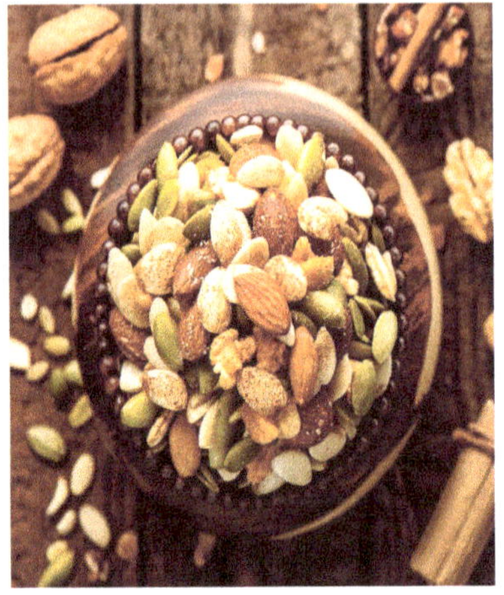

Preparation time: 10 minutes
Servings: 2-3

Ingredients:
- 1/2 cup rolled oats (gluten-free if needed)
- 1/4 cup pumpkin seeds
- 1/4 cup sunflower seeds
- **Optional additions (choose low-FODMAP options in limited amounts):**
 - Chopped dried fruit like cranberries or blueberries
 - Shredded unsweetened coconut
 - Chopped nuts like almonds or cashews

Directions:
1. In a large bowl, combine the rolled oats, pumpkin seeds, and sunflower seeds.

2. Stir in any additional low-FODMAP ingredients you like, such as chopped dried fruit, shredded coconut, or chopped nuts (be mindful of portion sizes due to FODMAP content in some nuts).

3. Mix everything well and store in an airtight container at room temperature for up to a week.

Nutritional value per serving (estimated - base recipe):

Calories: 250

Carbs: 30g

Cholesterol: 0mg

Total Fat: 10g

Fiber: 5g

Protein: 5g

Sodium: 30mg

Notes:

- Trail mix is a convenient and portable snack that is perfect for on-the-go situations.

- Feel free to customize the ingredients according to your preferences and what you have available. Just be sure to stick with low-FODMAP options and limit portion sizes of certain ingredients like nuts and dried fruits.

- This recipe is a starting point, feel free to get creative and add your favorite low-FODMAP flavors!

Roasted Chickpeas with Spices

Preparation time: 10 minutes
Cooking time: 40-45 minutes
Servings: 2-3

Ingredients:
- 1 (15 oz) can chickpeas, drained and rinsed
- 1 tablespoon olive oil
- 1/2 teaspoon ground cumin
- 1/4 teaspoon smoked paprika
- 1/4 teaspoon garlic powder
- Pinch of cayenne pepper (optional)
- Salt and black pepper to taste

Directions:
1. Preheat oven to 400°F (200°C). Line a baking sheet with parchment paper.
2. Pat the drained and rinsed chickpeas dry with a clean kitchen towel to remove any excess moisture. This will help them crisp up better in the oven.
3. In a large bowl, toss the chickpeas with olive oil, ground cumin, smoked paprika, garlic powder, and cayenne pepper (if using). Season with salt and black pepper to taste.

4. Spread the seasoned chickpeas in a single layer on the prepared baking sheet.

5. Roast the chickpeas for 30-35 minutes, stirring occasionally, until they are golden brown and crispy.

6. Remove the baking sheet from the oven and let the roasted chickpeas cool slightly before serving.

Nutritional value per serving (estimated):

Calories: 200
Carbs: 20g
Cholesterol: 0mg
Total Fat: 5g

Fiber: 5g
Protein: 10g
Sodium: 300mg

Notes:

- You can experiment with other low-FODMAP spices like ground coriander, turmeric, or nutritional yeast for different flavor variations.

- Roasted chickpeas are a delicious and healthy snack or can be added to salads, bowls, or wraps for extra protein and crunch.

- Leftover roasted chickpeas can be stored in an airtight container at room temperature for up to 3 days or in the refrigerator for up to a week.

Coconut Chia Seed Pudding

Preparation time: 5 minutes | Servings: 1

Ingredients:
- 1/3 cup unsweetened almond milk or coconut milk (choose a low-FODMAP brand)
- 2 tablespoons chia seeds
- 1/4 teaspoon ground vanilla powder (optional)
- Pinch of ground cinnamon
- **Toppings (optional)**:
  - Chopped fresh fruit (low-FODMAP options like berries)
  - Shredded unsweetened coconut
  - A drizzle of maple syrup (limited amount due to FODMAP content)

Directions:

1. In a small jar or container, combine the unsweetened almond milk (or coconut milk), chia seeds, vanilla powder (if using), and ground cinnamon.

2. Mix thoroughly to ensure all the ingredients are well combined.

3. Cover the jar or container and refrigerate for at least 4 hours, or preferably overnight, to allow the chia seeds to absorb the liquid and thicken into a pudding consistency.

4. In the morning, stir the pudding again before serving.

Serving Suggestions:
- Top the chia seed pudding with your favorite low-FODMAP chopped fresh fruits like berries, shredded unsweetened coconut, or a drizzle of maple syrup (limited amount).
- You can enjoy this pudding for breakfast, a snack, or even a light dessert.

Nutritional value per serving (estimated - base recipe):

Calories: 150   *Fiber: 5g*
Carbs: 15g   *Protein: 2g*
Cholesterol: 0mg   *Sodium: 10mg*
Total Fat: 5g

Notes:
- Feel free to adjust the amount of chia seeds depending on how thick you like your pudding.
- You can add a pinch of ground ginger or nutmeg for a different flavor twist.
- Leftover chia seed pudding can be stored in an airtight container in the refrigerator for up to 3 days.

Baked Sweet Potato Fries

*Preparation time: 10 minutes | Cooking time:
20-25 minutes | Servings: 2-3*

Ingredients:
- 1 large sweet potato
- 1 tablespoon olive oil
- 1/2 teaspoon ground paprika
- 1/4 teaspoon garlic powder
- Salt and black pepper to taste

Directions:
1. Preheat oven to 400°F (200°C). Place parchment paper on a baking sheet.
2. Wash and dry the sweet potato. Peel it if desired, or leave the skin on for added nutrients. Slice the sweet potato into thin sticks, about ¼ inch thick and ¼ inch wide. Try to achieve a consistent thickness to ensure even cooking.
3. In a large bowl, toss the sweet potato sticks with olive oil, paprika, garlic powder, salt, and black pepper. Ensure that the spices are evenly spread throughout the mixture.
4. Spread the seasoned sweet potato fries in a single layer on the prepared baking sheet, ensuring they are not touching or overlapping. Overcrowding can prevent them from crisping up properly.
5. Bake the sweet potato fries for 20-25 minutes, or until tender on the inside and golden brown and

crispy on the outside. Flip the fries halfway through baking for even browning.

6. Remove the baking sheet from the oven and let the fries cool slightly before serving. Enjoy them plain or with your favorite dipping sauces like ketchup (check for low-FODMAP options) or a simple mixture of olive oil and herbs.

Nutritional value per serving (estimated):

Calories: 200   *Fiber: 4g*
Carbs: 25g   *Protein: 1g*
Cholesterol: 0mg   *Sodium: 60mg*
Total Fat: 5g

Notes:
- You can experiment with other low-FODMAP spices like ground cumin, turmeric, or nutritional yeast for different flavor variations.
- For extra crispy fries, soak the sliced sweet potatoes in cold water for 30 minutes before tossing them with the spices and baking. This helps to remove some of the starch, which can prevent them from crisping up properly.
- You can store leftover baked sweet potato fries in an airtight container in the refrigerator for up to 3 days. Reheat them in the oven or toaster oven before serving.

Fruit and Vegetable Smoothie

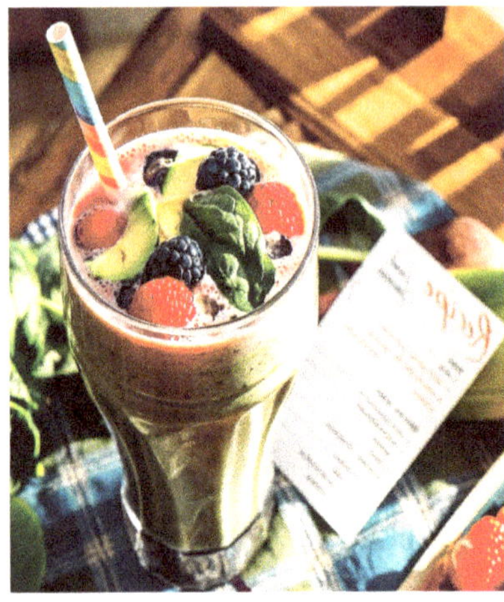

Preparation time:
5 minutes
Servings: 1

Ingredients:
- 1 cup unsweetened almond milk or coconut milk (choose a low-FODMAP brand)
- ½ cup frozen low-FODMAP fruits (e.g., berries, kiwi, peeled pineapple)
- ½ cup chopped low-FODMAP vegetables (e.g., spinach, cucumber, zucchini)
- 1 tablespoon ground flaxseed meal (optional)
- Pinch of ground cinnamon (optional)

Directions:
1. In a blender, combine the unsweetened almond milk (or coconut milk), frozen fruits, chopped

vegetables, ground flaxseed meal (if using), and ground cinnamon (if using).

2. Blend until smooth and creamy. You may need to add a little more liquid if the mixture is too thick.

3. Transfer the smoothie into a glass and savor it!

Nutritional value per serving (estimated):

Calories: 200

Carbs: 30g

Cholesterol: 0mg

Total Fat: 5g

Fiber: 5g

Protein: 2g

Sodium: 10mg

Notes:

- Feel free to experiment with different combinations of low-FODMAP fruits and vegetables to create your own favorite flavor variations.

- You can add a scoop of low-FODMAP protein powder for an extra protein boost.

- Leftover smoothie can be stored in an airtight container in the refrigerator for up to 1 day, but the taste and texture may be slightly altered.

No-Bake Energy Bites

Preparation time: 15 minutes | Chilling time: At least 30 minutes | Servings: 10-12 bites

Ingredients:
- ½ cup rolled oats (gluten-free if needed)
- ¼ cup unsweetened shredded coconut
- ¼ cup chopped pitted dates
- ¼ cup almond butter (check for low-FODMAP options)
- 2 tablespoons chia seeds
- 2 tablespoons ground flaxseed meal
- Pinch of ground cinnamon
- **Optional additions (in very limited amounts due to FODMAP content):**
    - Chopped nuts (cashews or almonds)
    - Dried fruit (chopped cranberries or blueberries)

Directions:
1. In a large bowl, combine the rolled oats, shredded coconut, chopped dates, almond butter, chia seeds, ground flaxseed meal, and ground cinnamon.
2. Mix well until all the ingredients are well combined and the mixture sticks together easily.
3. If the mixture feels too dry, add a tablespoon of water or unsweetened almond milk at a time until it reaches a consistency that can be easily formed into balls.

4. Fold in any optional chopped nuts or dried fruit (be mindful of portion sizes).

5. Using a spoon or your hands, roll the mixture into small balls, about 1 inch in diameter.

6. Arrange the energy bites on a baking sheet that's lined with parchment paper..

7. Refrigerate the energy bites for at least 30 minutes, or until they are firm and set.

Nutritional value per serving (estimated - base recipe):

Calories: 150
Carbs: 20g
Cholesterol: 0mg
Total Fat: 5g

Fiber: 5g
Protein: 3g
Sodium: 30mg

Notes:
- These no-bake energy bites are a convenient and portable snack that is perfect for on-the-go situations.
- You can adjust the ingredients and flavors to your preference. Just be sure to stick with low-FODMAP options and limit portion sizes of certain ingredients.
- Leftover energy bites can be stored in an airtight container in the refrigerator for up to a week.

Homemade Vegan Yogurt with Berries

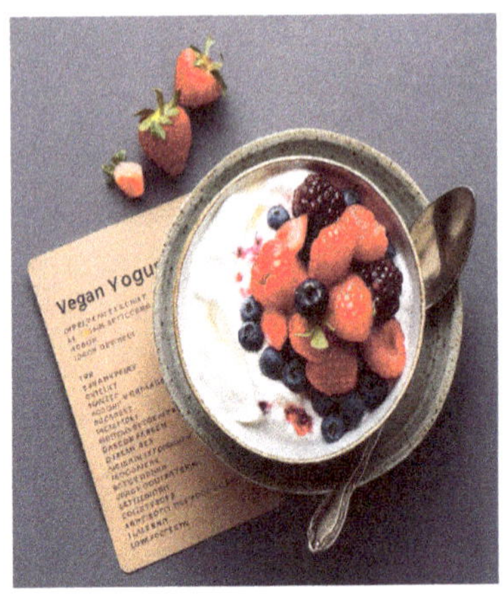

Preparation time: 10 minutes (plus overnight incubation)
Servings: 1-2

Ingredients:

- 1 cup unsweetened almond milk or coconut milk (choose a low-FODMAP brand)
- 2 tablespoons vegan yogurt starter with live and active cultures (check for low-FODMAP options)
- ¼ cup frozen low-FODMAP berries (e.g., blueberries, raspberries) - for topping (optional)

Directions:

1. In a small saucepan, heat the unsweetened almond milk (or coconut milk) over low heat until lukewarm (around 105°F /41°C). Do not let the milk boil.

2. **Important**: Turn off the heat and let the milk cool slightly if it exceeds 105°F (41°C). The temperature needs to be lukewarm but not hot, as excessively high temperatures can kill the live and active cultures in the yogurt starter.

3. Pour the lukewarm milk into a clean jar or container. Stir in the vegan yogurt starter with live and active cultures until well combined.

4. Cover the jar or container tightly with a lid. Wrap the jar or container in a clean kitchen towel or blanket to help insulate it and maintain warmth.

5. Place the jar or container in a warm location, ideally around 100°F (38°C) for 8-10 hours, or overnight. You can achieve this by placing it near a warm appliance (not directly touching) or using a yogurt maker (if you have one).

6. After incubation, check the consistency of the yogurt. It should be thickened and set. If it is still too runny, let it incubate for a few more hours.

7. Refrigerate the homemade vegan yogurt for at least 2 hours to allow it to chill and further thicken.

8. Serve the chilled yogurt plain or topped with your favorite low-FODMAP frozen berries (limited amount) or other toppings like chopped nuts (limited amount) and shredded unsweetened coconut.

Nutritional value per serving (estimated - base recipe):

Calories: 150
Carbs: 15g
Cholesterol: 0mg
Total Fat: 5g

Fiber: 1g
Protein: 2g
Sodium: 10mg

Notes:

- It is important to use a vegan yogurt starter with live and active cultures specifically labeled as low-FODMAP. Not all vegan yogurt starters are created equal, and some may contain high-FODMAP ingredients.

- The temperature during incubation is crucial for successful yogurt fermentation. If the milk is too cold, the cultures may not activate properly. If the milk is too hot, it can kill the cultures.

- You can reuse a portion of your homemade yogurt as a starter for your next batch, as long as it is fresh and within a week of making it.

Chapter 7: Conversion Charts & Glossary

This bonus chapter equips you with helpful tools to navigate the world of vegan SIBO management and understand the recipes in this book.

Conversion Charts

Baking and cooking often require precise measurements. Here's a guide to convert between common units:

- **1 cup (US) equals 240 milliliters (ml).**
- **1 tablespoon (US) equals 15 milliliters (ml).**
- **1 teaspoon (US) equals 5 milliliters (ml).**
- **1 pound equals 453.6 grams (g).**
- **1 ounce equals 28.3 grams (g).**
- **1 inch equals 2.54 centimeters (cm).**

Glossary

- **Bloating**: A feeling of abdominal distention caused by gas buildup in the digestive system.
- **Constipation**: Difficulty passing stool infrequently or with difficulty.

- **Diarrhea:** Loose, watery stools that happen more often than usual.
- **Elimination Diet**: A dietary approach where certain foods are temporarily removed to identify triggers for digestive issues.
- **Fermentable Oligosaccharides, Disaccharides, Monosaccharides, and Polyols (FODMAPs)**: Short-chain carbohydrates that can be poorly absorbed in the small intestine and contribute to digestive problems.
- **Gut Microbiome**: The community of microorganisms (bacteria, fungi, etc.) residing in the gut, playing a crucial role in digestion, immune function, and overall health.
- **IBS (Irritable Bowel Syndrome)**: A chronic condition characterized by abdominal pain, cramping, bloating, diarrhea, and constipation.
- **Inflammation**: The body's natural response to injury or infection, but chronic inflammation can contribute to various health problems.
- **Intestinal Lining**: The inner layer of the small intestine responsible for nutrient absorption.
- **Low-FODMAP Diet:** A structured elimination and reintroduction approach

designed to identify and manage food intolerances related to FODMAPs.

- **Micronutrients**: Essential vitamins and minerals required in small amounts for various bodily functions.
- **Nutrient Absorption**: The process by which nutrients from food are taken up by the body through the digestive system.
- **Prebiotics**: Non-digestible fibers that act as food for beneficial bacteria in the gut, helping them grow and thrive.
- **Probiotics**: Live bacteria that provide health benefits by promoting a healthy gut microbiome.
- **Registered Dietitian (RD):** A qualified healthcare professional specializing in dietary and nutritional counseling.
- **SIBO (Small Intestinal Bacterial Overgrowth):** A condition where there's an abnormal rise in the quantity and/or variety of bacteria in the small intestine.
- **Symptoms**: Physical or mental experiences that indicate a disease or condition.

Additional Resources

* Websites of reputable health organizations like the National Institutes of Health (NIH) or the International Foundation for Functional Gastrointestinal Disorders (IFFGD) can provide further information on SIBO and the low-FODMAP diet.
* Consider joining online communities or support groups focused on vegan diets or SIBO management to connect with others on a similar journey.

We hope this bonus chapter aids you in your exploration of vegan SIBO management. Remember, this information is intended for educational purposes only and does not substitute for professional medical advice. Consult a healthcare professional for personalized guidance on managing SIBO and creating a diet plan that aligns with your specific needs.

14-Day Vegan SIBO-Friendly Meal Plan

Day 1:
Breakfast: Chia Seed Pudding
Lunch: Vegetable Curry with Quinoa
Dinner: Stir-Fried Noodles with Tofu
Snack: Baked Apple with Cinnamon and Walnuts

Day 2:
Breakfast: Buckwheat Pancakes
Lunch: Lentil Soup
Dinner: Thai Green Curry with Vegetables
Snack: Homemade Rice Cakes with Guacamole

Day 3:
Breakfast: Coconut Yogurt Parfait
Lunch: Coconut Curry Noodle Bowl
Dinner: Vegan Chili
Snack: Frozen Banana Bites

Day 4:
Breakfast: Vegetable Frittata
Lunch: Stuffed Portobello Mushrooms
Dinner: Stuffed Sweet Potatoes
Snack: Trail Mix with Nuts and Seeds

<table>
<tr><td>

Day 5:

Breakfast: Green Smoothie

Lunch: Rainbow Veggie Wraps

Dinner: Lentil Shepherd's Pie

Snack: Roasted Chickpeas with Spices

</td><td>

Day 6:

Breakfast: Tofu Scramble

Lunch: Edamame Salad with Quinoa

Dinner: Coconut Curry Lentil Soup

Snack: Coconut Chia Seed Pudding

</td></tr>
<tr><td>

Day 7:

Breakfast: Seaweed Salad

Lunch: Vegetable Skewers with Tahini Dip

Dinner: Vegan Paella

Snack: Baked Sweet Potato Fries

</td><td>

Day 8:

Breakfast: Roasted Sweet Potato Toast

Lunch: Quinoa Buddha Bowl

Dinner: Vegetable Fajitas

Snack: Fruit and Vegetable Smoothie

</td></tr>
</table>

Day 9:

Breakfast: Savory Chickpea Scramble
Lunch: Vegetable Curry with Quinoa
Dinner: Stir-Fried Noodles with Tofu
Snack: Baked Apple with Cinnamon and Walnuts

Day 10:

Breakfast: Savory Chickpea Scramble
Lunch: Lentil Soup
Dinner: Thai Green Curry with Vegetables
Snack: Homemade Vegan Yogurt with Berries

Day 11:

Breakfast: Green Smoothie
Lunch: Edamame Salad with Quinoa
Dinner: Coconut Curry Lentil Soup
Snack: Coconut Chia Seed Pudding

Day 12:

Breakfast: Seaweed Salad
Lunch: Quinoa Buddha Bowl
Dinner: Vegetable Fajitas
Snack: Fruit and Vegetable Smoothie

<table>
<tr><td>

Day 13:
Breakfast: Sprouted Lentil Breakfast Bowl
Lunch: Coconut Curry Chickpea Salad Sandwich
Dinner: Coconut Curry Chickpea Bowls
Snack: Homemade Vegan Yogurt with Berries

</td><td>

Day 14:
Breakfast: Buckwheat Pancakes
Lunch: Coconut Curry Noodle Bowl
Dinner: Vegan Chili
Snack: Frozen Banana Bites

</td></tr>
</table>

Notes:

- This is a sample meal plan, feel free to adjust it based on your preferences and the availability of ingredients.
- Leftovers can be used for lunch or dinner the next day.
- Be sure to drink plenty of water throughout the day.
- You can add low-FODMAP herbs and spices to your meals for additional flavor.

Enjoy your delicious and gut-friendly meals!

Conclusion

You've reached the end of your journey through the delicious world of vegan SIBO-friendly recipes! Hopefully, Uncle Peter's story and the exploration of gut-friendly meals have left you feeling empowered and inspired. But remember, this is just the starting point.

Consider this book your culinary compass, guiding you towards a future filled with vibrant flavors and a happy gut. As you navigate these recipes, feel free to experiment! Swap in your favorite low-FODMAP ingredients, adjust spice levels to your preference, and unleash your inner culinary genius. After all, a healthy gut shouldn't come at the expense of flavor exploration.

Remember, managing SIBO is a marathon, not a sprint. There will be days when cravings tempt you, and social situations feel like minefields of potential digestive triggers. That's okay! This book is here to be your trusted companion, offering a delicious and safe haven whenever you need it.

Most importantly, don't be afraid to listen to your body. SIBO can manifest differently in everyone, so pay attention to how certain ingredients affect you. Use the low-FODMAP framework as a guide, but personalize it to create a long-term eating plan that works for you.

As you embark on this journey, remember the power of a positive mindset. Focus on the incredible things a well-nourished gut can do for you – increased energy, clearer thinking, and a happier disposition. Celebrate your non-bloated victories, no matter how small they seem.

Finally, share your success story! This invisible enemy called SIBO can feel isolating. But by sharing your journey with others, you can inspire them to take control of their gut health and embrace a delicious, plant-based lifestyle. So, spread the word, host low-FODMAP potlucks, and let's create a community that thrives on gut health and culinary adventures.

This book is more than just a collection of recipes; it's a starting point for a healthier, happier you. So, keep exploring, keep experimenting, and most importantly, keep feeling fantastic!

Weekly Meal Planner

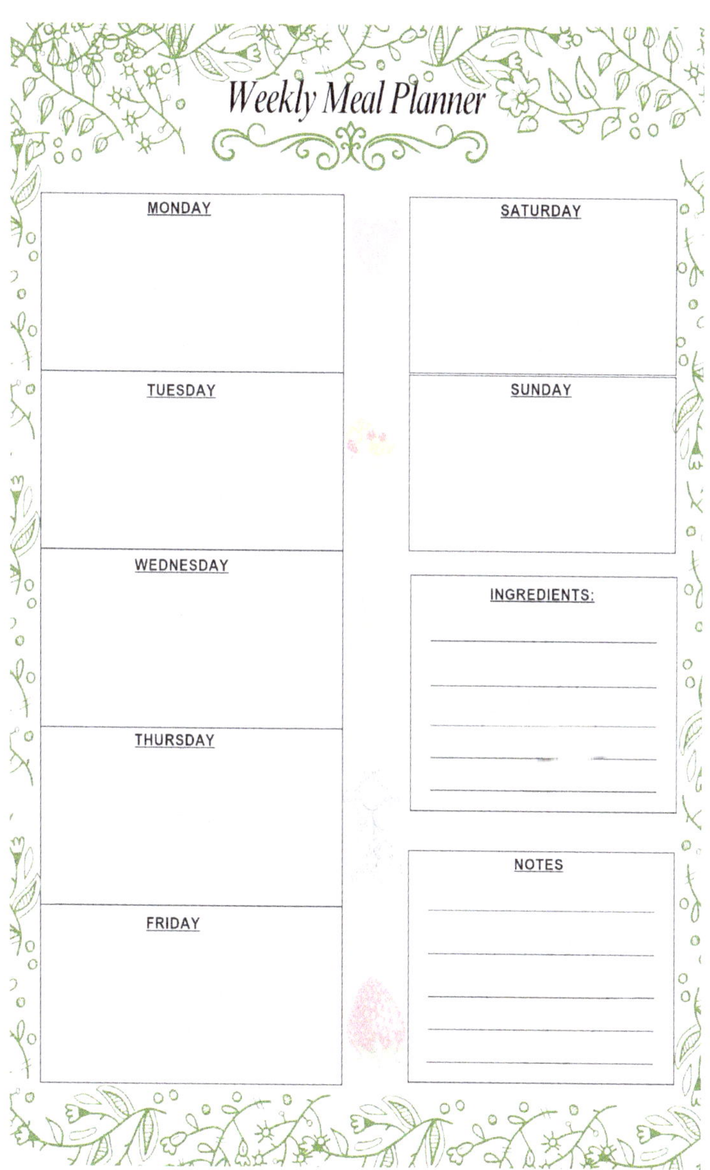

Weekly Meal Planner

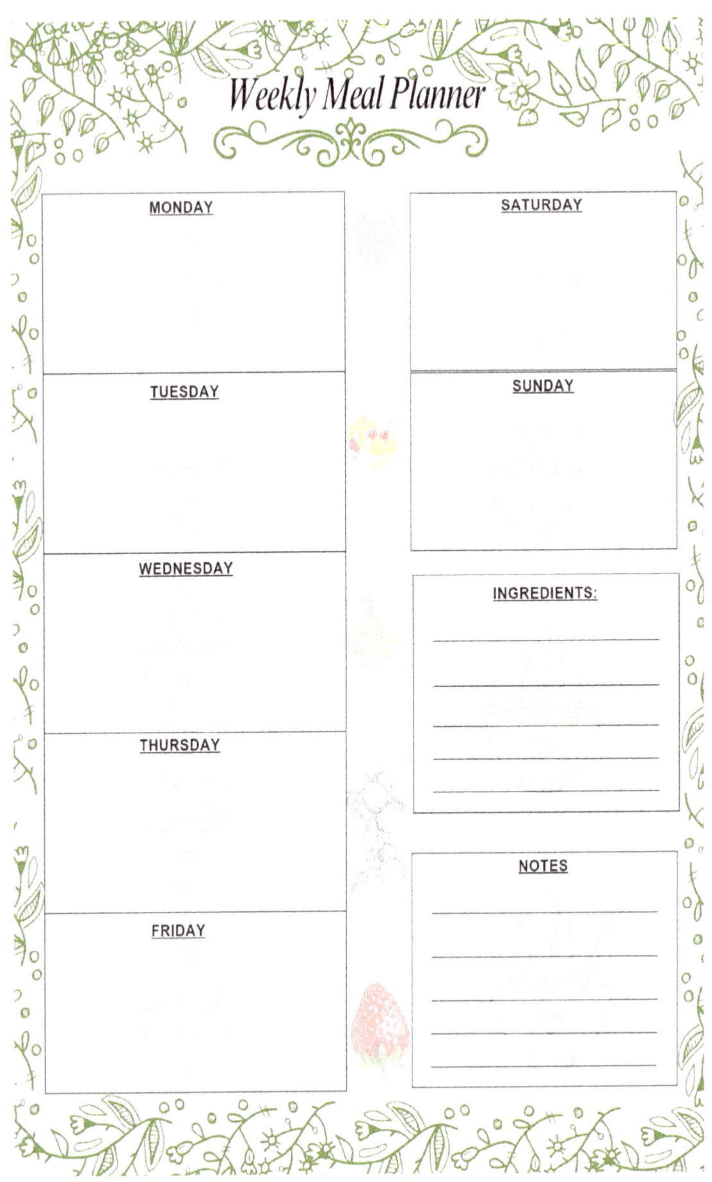

MONDAY	SATURDAY
TUESDAY	SUNDAY
WEDNESDAY	INGREDIENTS:
THURSDAY	
FRIDAY	NOTES

Weekly Meal Planner

MONDAY

TUESDAY

WEDNESDAY

THURSDAY

FRIDAY

SATURDAY

SUNDAY

INGREDIENTS:

NOTES

Weekly Meal Planner

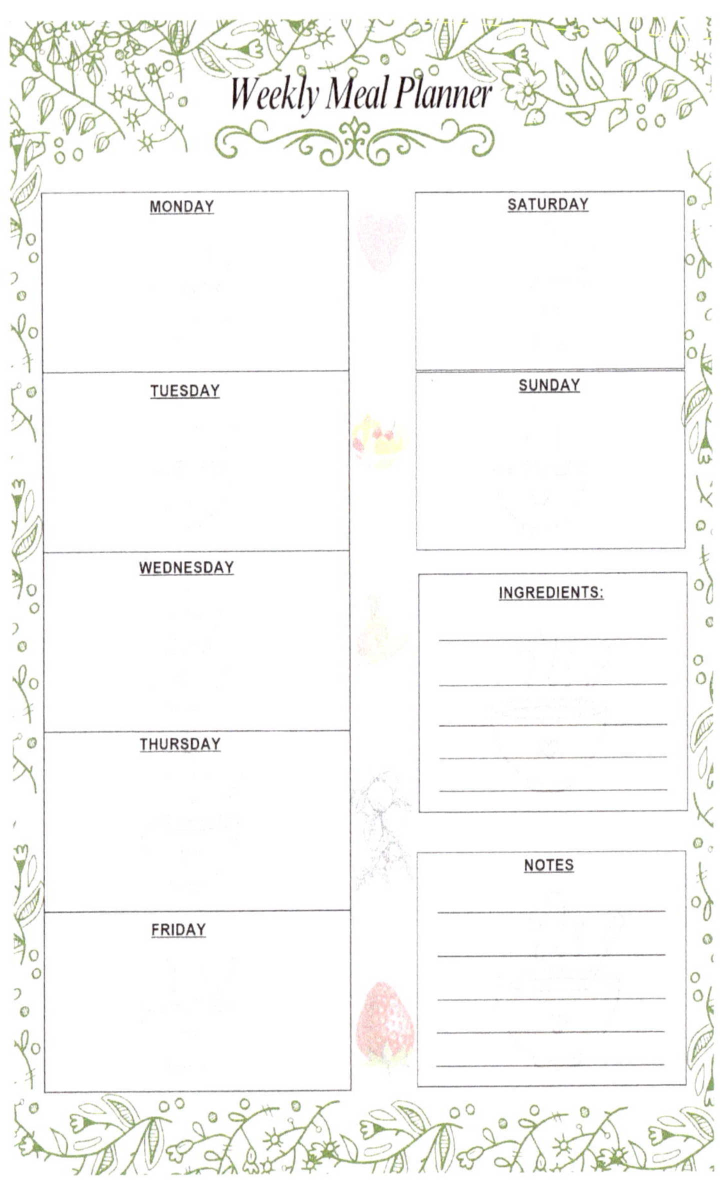

Weekly Meal Planner

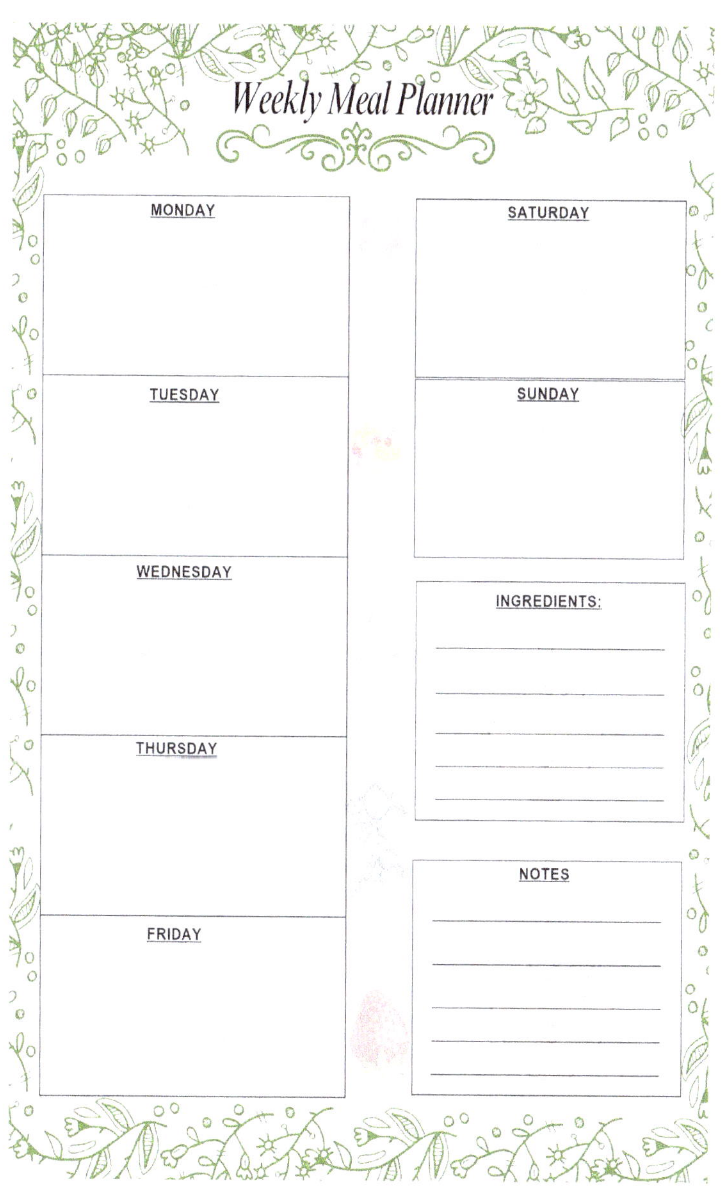

Weekly Meal Planner

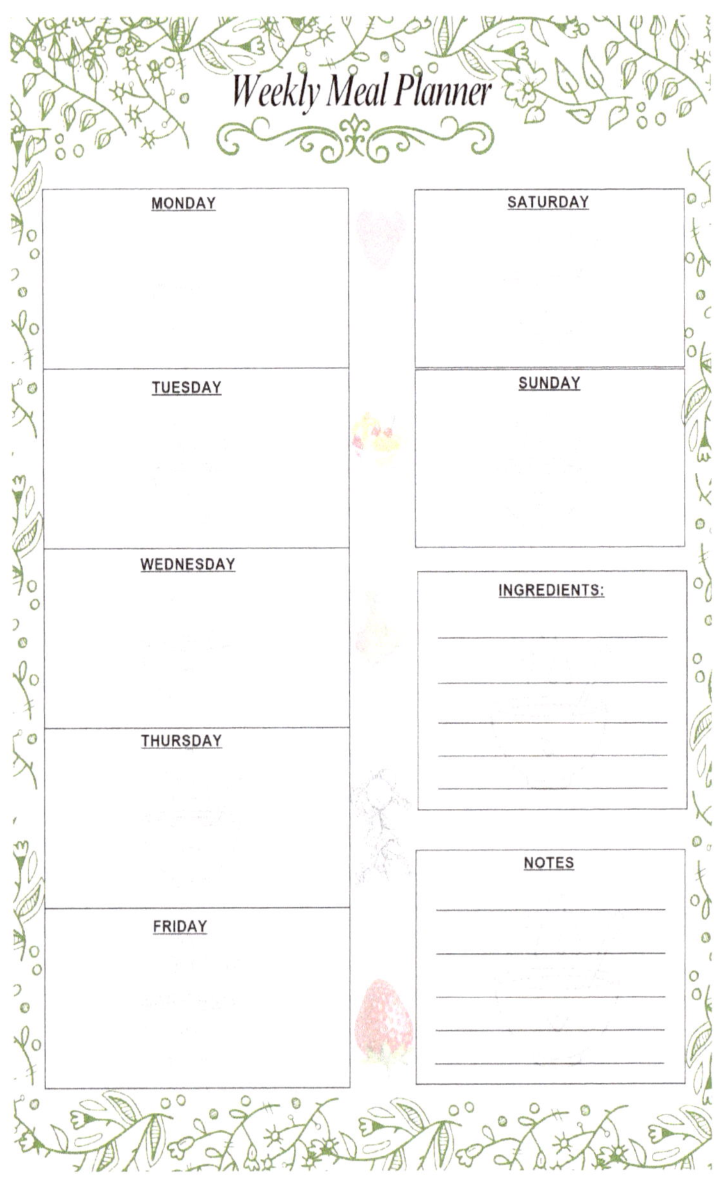

Weekly Meal Planner

MONDAY

SATURDAY

TUESDAY

SUNDAY

WEDNESDAY

INGREDIENTS:

THURSDAY

FRIDAY

NOTES

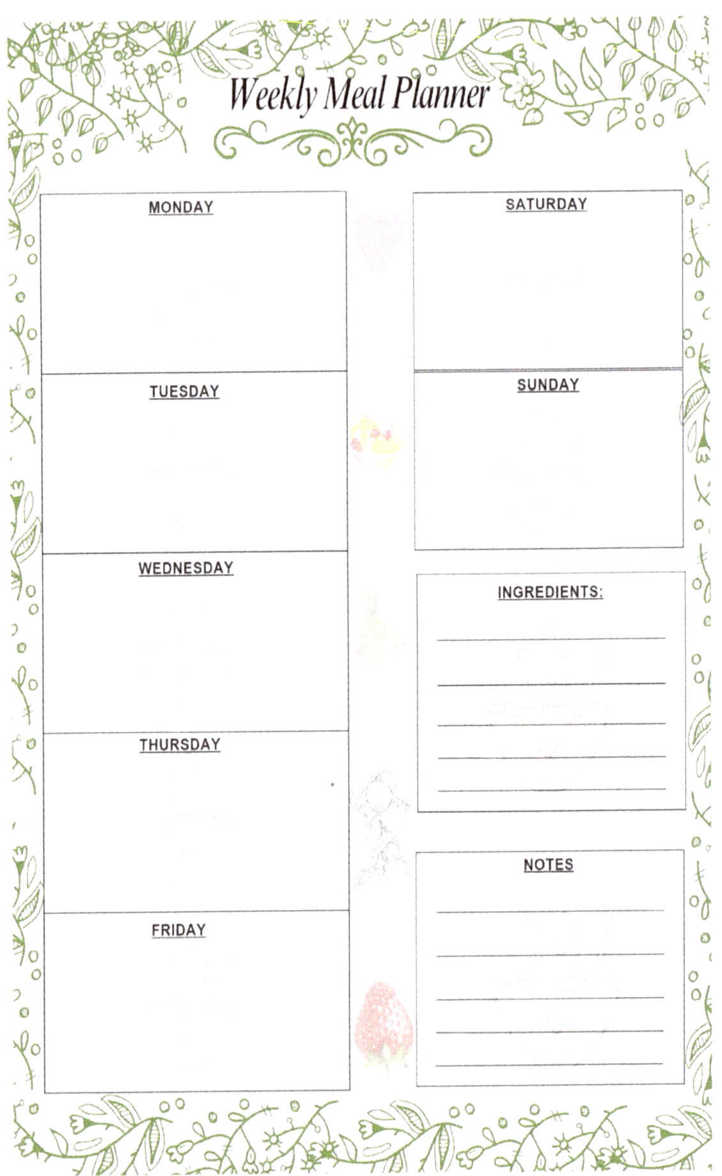

Weekly Meal Planner
MONDAY
TUESDAY
WEDNESDAY
THURSDAY
FRIDAY
SATURDAY
SUNDAY
INGREDIENTS:
NOTES

Weekly Meal Planner

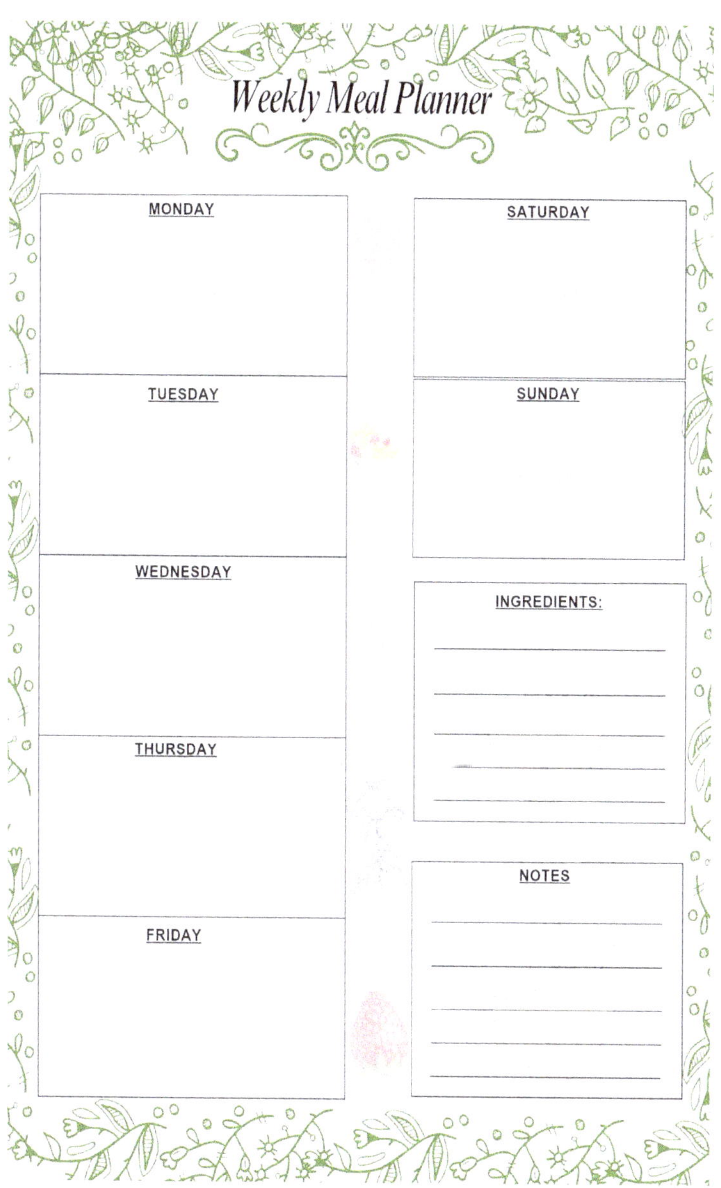

Weekly Meal Planner

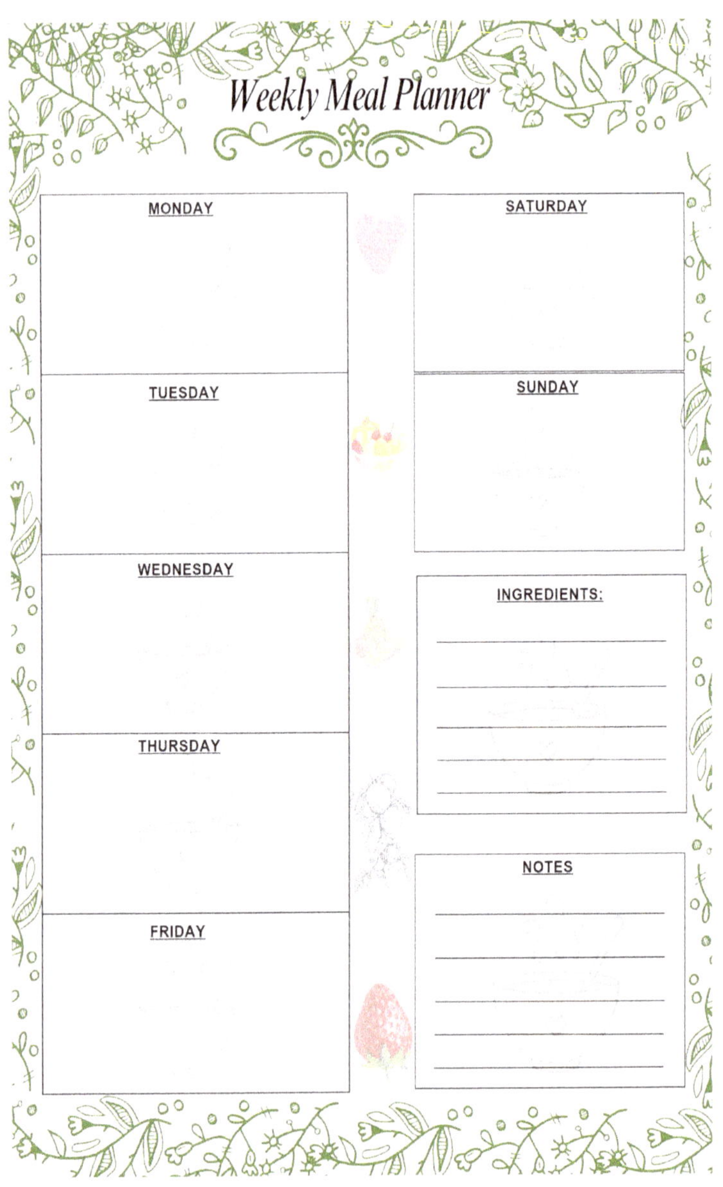

MONDAY

TUESDAY

WEDNESDAY

THURSDAY

FRIDAY

SATURDAY

SUNDAY

INGREDIENTS:

NOTES

Weekly Meal Planner

MONDAY

TUESDAY

WEDNESDAY

THURSDAY

FRIDAY

SATURDAY

SUNDAY

INGREDIENTS:

NOTES

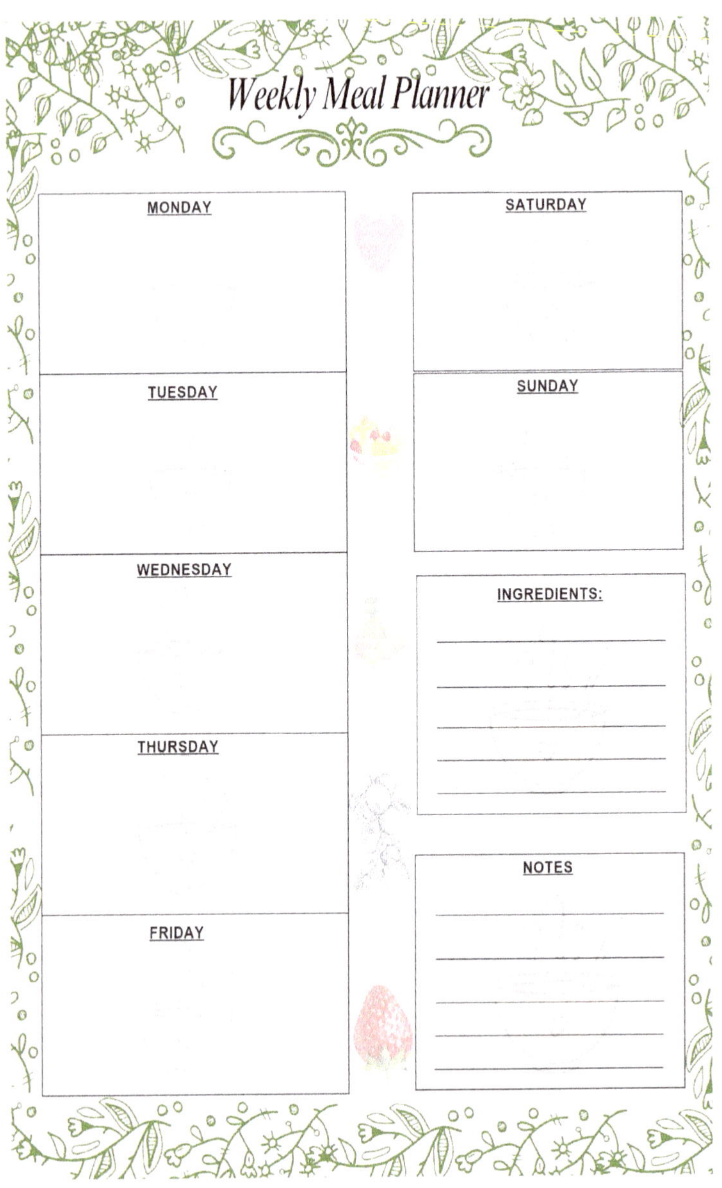

Weekly Meal Planner
MONDAY
TUESDAY
WEDNESDAY
THURSDAY
FRIDAY
SATURDAY
SUNDAY
INGREDIENTS:
NOTES

Weekly Meal Planner

MONDAY

TUESDAY

WEDNESDAY

THURSDAY

FRIDAY

SATURDAY

SUNDAY

INGREDIENTS:

NOTES

Weekly Meal Planner

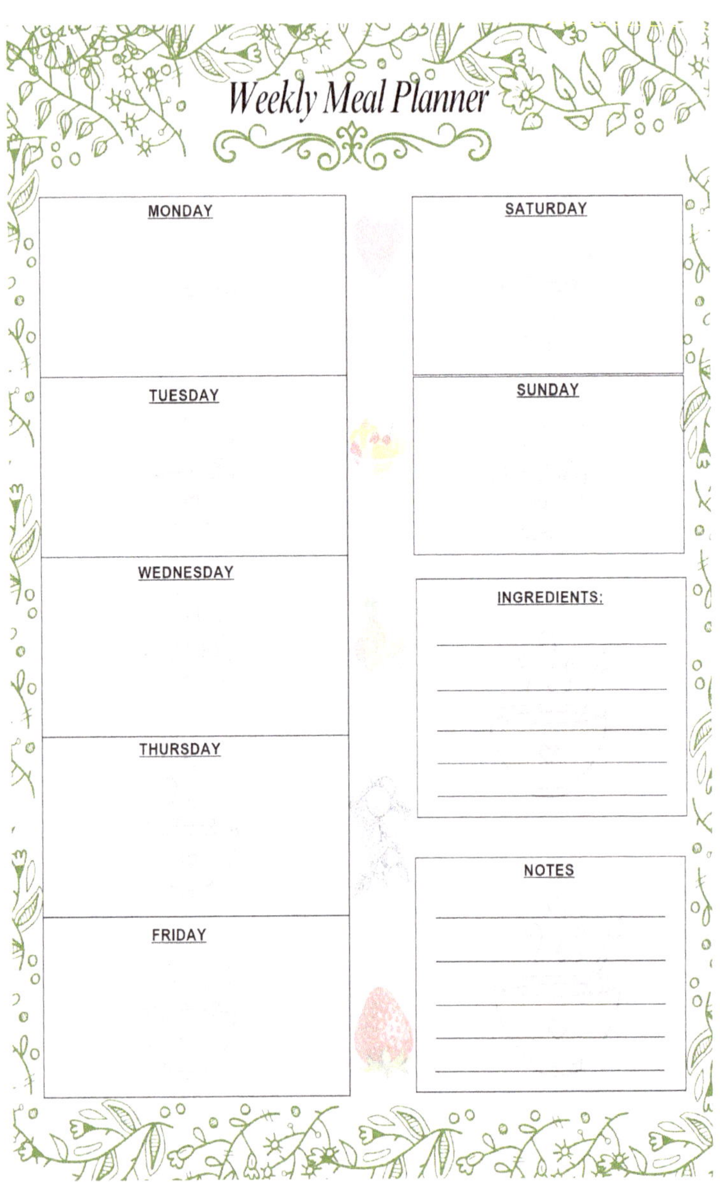

MONDAY	**SATURDAY**
TUESDAY	**SUNDAY**
WEDNESDAY	**INGREDIENTS:**
THURSDAY	
FRIDAY	**NOTES**

Weekly Meal Planner

MONDAY

TUESDAY

WEDNESDAY

THURSDAY

FRIDAY

SATURDAY

SUNDAY

INGREDIENTS:

NOTES

Weekly Meal Planner

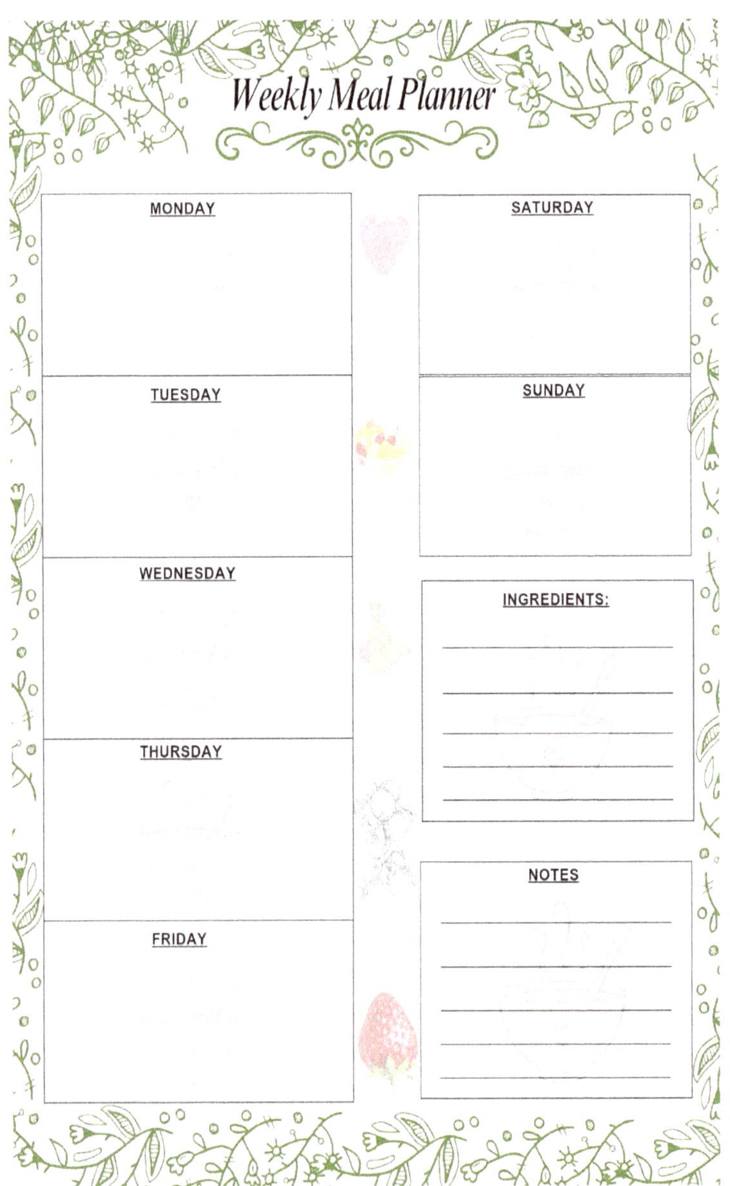

Weekly Meal Planner

MONDAY

TUESDAY

WEDNESDAY

THURSDAY

FRIDAY

SATURDAY

SUNDAY

INGREDIENTS:

NOTES

Weekly Meal Planner

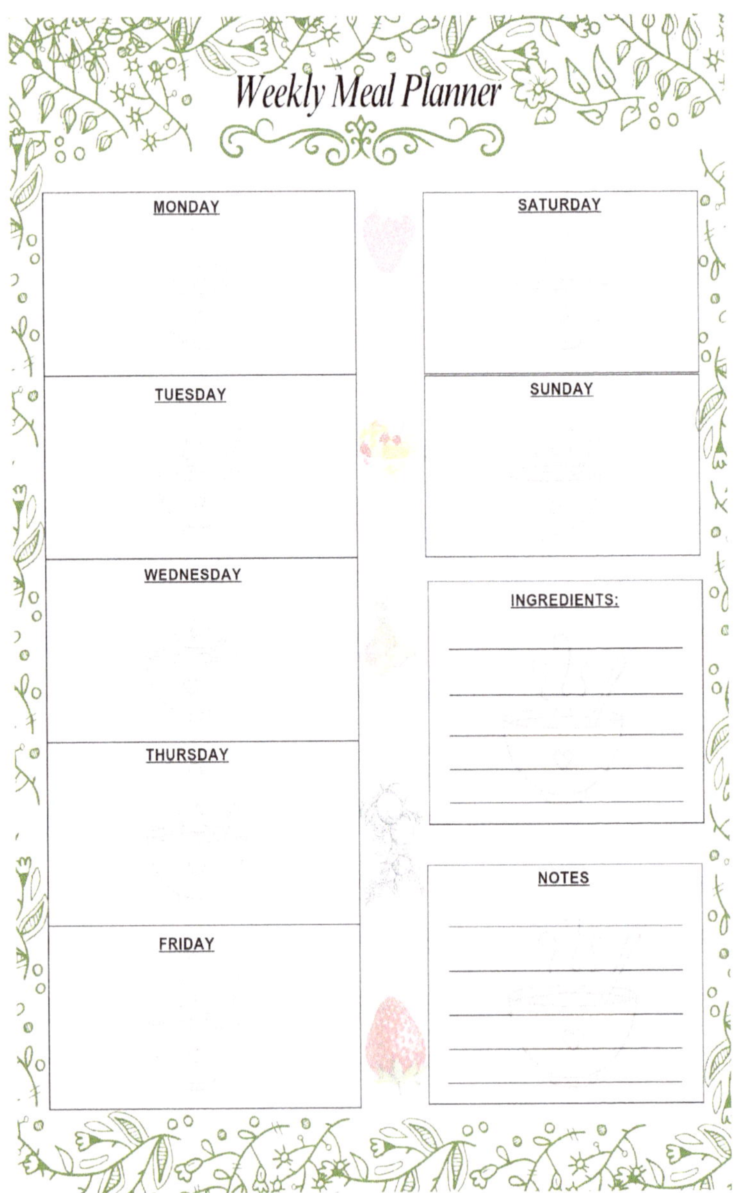

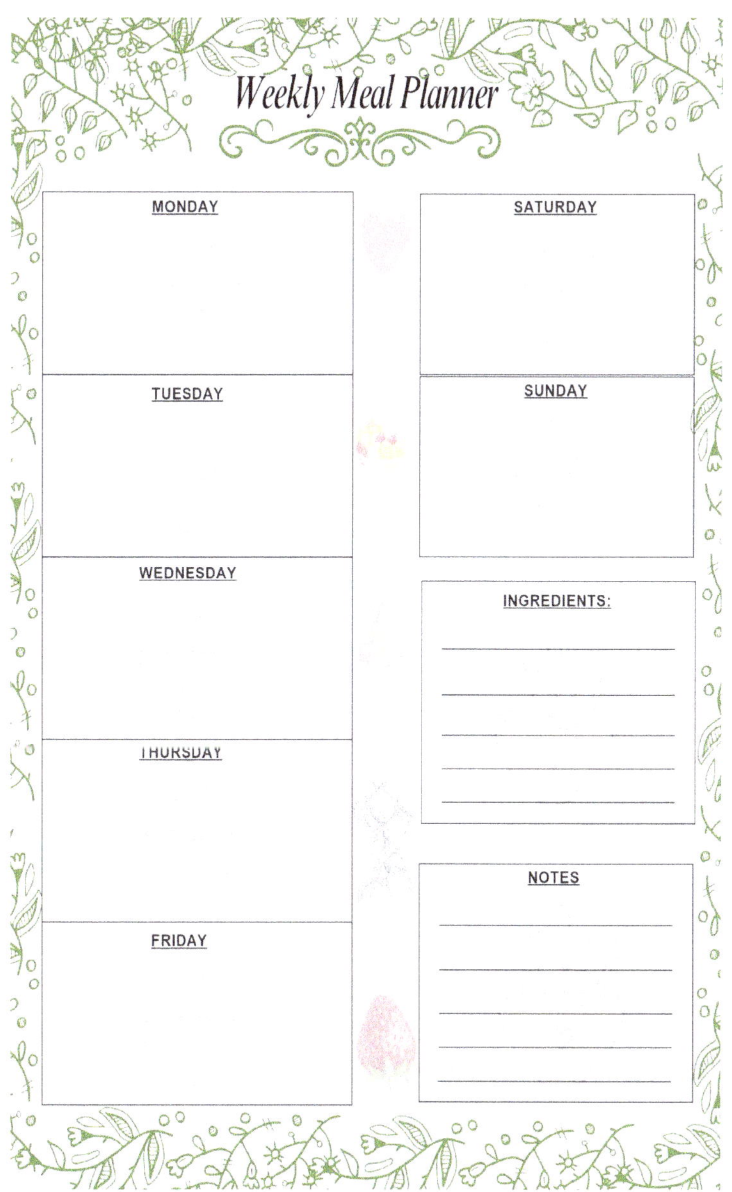

Weekly Meal Planner
MONDAY
TUESDAY
WEDNESDAY
THURSDAY
FRIDAY
SATURDAY
SUNDAY
INGREDIENTS:
NOTES

Weekly Meal Planner

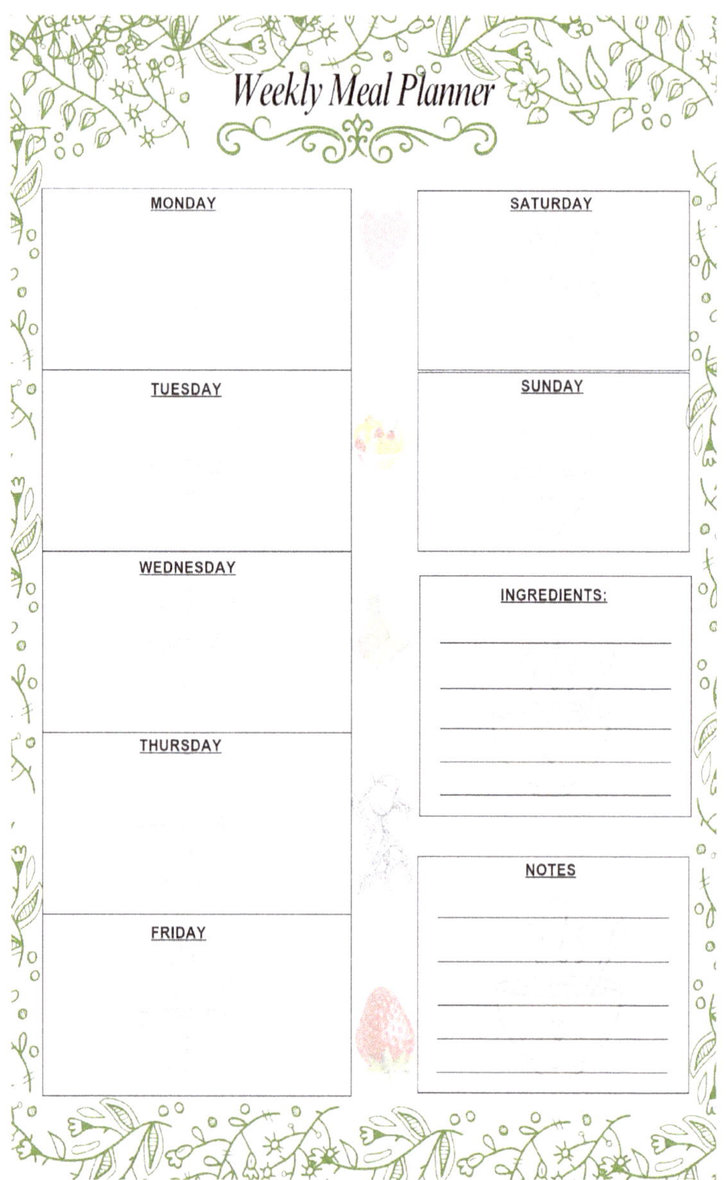

MONDAY	SATURDAY
TUESDAY	SUNDAY
WEDNESDAY	INGREDIENTS:
THURSDAY	NOTES
FRIDAY	

Weekly Meal Planner

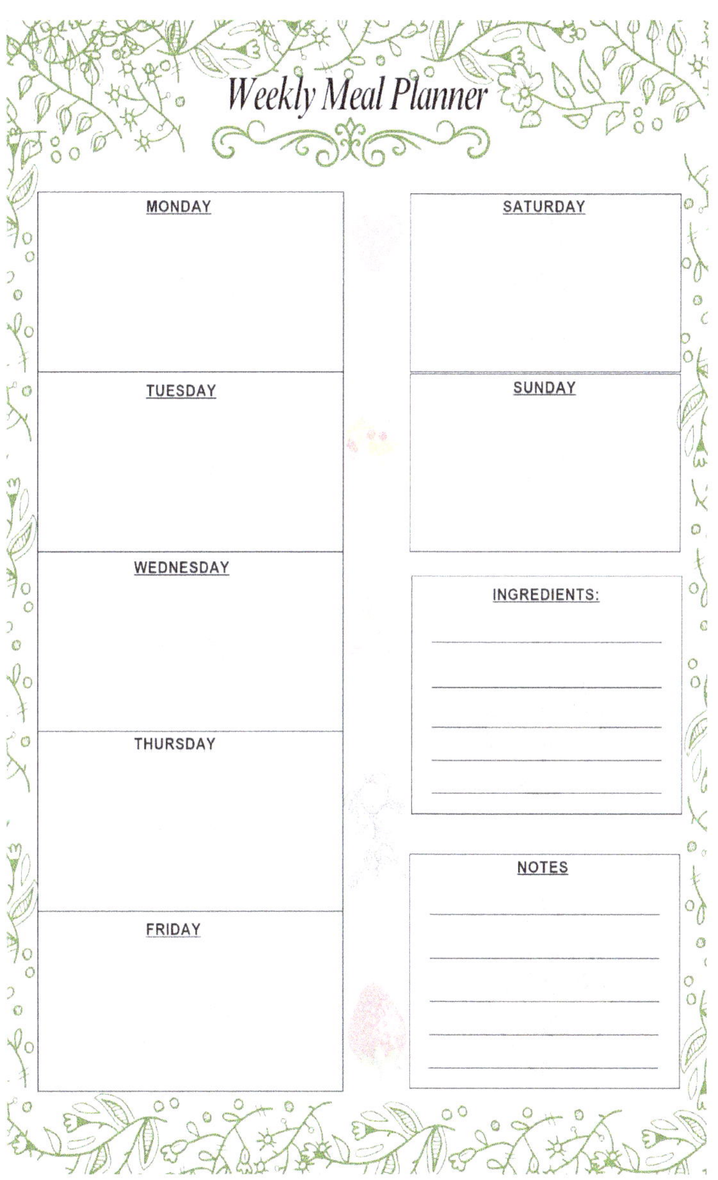

www.ingramcontent.com/pod-product-compliance
Lightning Source LLC
Chambersburg PA
CBHW071012250726
48653CB00005B/1590